NURSING - ISSUES, PROBLEMS AND CHALLENGES

U.S. NURSING WORKFORCE

SUPPLY AND EDUCATION TRENDS

Nursing - Issues, Problems and Challenges

Additional books in this series can be found on Nova's website under the Series tab.

Additional e-books in this series can be found on Nova's website under the e-book tab.

NURSING - ISSUES, PROBLEMS AND CHALLENGES

U.S. NURSING WORKFORCE SUPPLY AND EDUCATION TRENDS

MARLA PARRIS
EDITOR

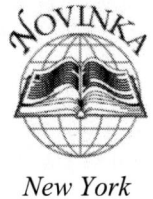

New York

Copyright © 2015 by Nova Science Publishers, Inc.

All rights reserved. No part of this book may be reproduced, stored in a retrieval system or transmitted in any form or by any means: electronic, electrostatic, magnetic, tape, mechanical photocopying, recording or otherwise without the written permission of the Publisher.

For permission to use material from this book please contact us:
nova.main@novapublishers.com

NOTICE TO THE READER

The Publisher has taken reasonable care in the preparation of this book, but makes no expressed or implied warranty of any kind and assumes no responsibility for any errors or omissions. No liability is assumed for incidental or consequential damages in connection with or arising out of information contained in this book. The Publisher shall not be liable for any special, consequential, or exemplary damages resulting, in whole or in part, from the readers' use of, or reliance upon, this material. Any parts of this book based on government reports are so indicated and copyright is claimed for those parts to the extent applicable to compilations of such works.

Independent verification should be sought for any data, advice or recommendations contained in this book. In addition, no responsibility is assumed by the publisher for any injury and/or damage to persons or property arising from any methods, products, instructions, ideas or otherwise contained in this publication.

This publication is designed to provide accurate and authoritative information with regard to the subject matter covered herein. It is sold with the clear understanding that the Publisher is not engaged in rendering legal or any other professional services. If legal or any other expert assistance is required, the services of a competent person should be sought. FROM A DECLARATION OF PARTICIPANTS JOINTLY ADOPTED BY A COMMITTEE OF THE AMERICAN BAR ASSOCIATION AND A COMMITTEE OF PUBLISHERS.

Additional color graphics may be available in the e-book version of this book.

Library of Congress Cataloging-in-Publication Data

ISBN: 978-1-63463-540-0

Published by Nova Science Publishers, Inc. † New York

CONTENTS

Preface		vii
Chapter 1	The U.S. Nursing Workforce: Trends in Supply and Education *National Center for Health Workforce Analysis*	1
Chapter 2	The U.S. Nursing Workforce: Technical Documentation *National Center for Health Workforce Analysis*	59
Index		65

PREFACE

This book analyzes data from a variety of sources to present recent trends and the current status of the registered nurse (RN) and licensed practical nurse (LPN) workforces. This book also provides additional information on data and methodology for analysis of the nurse supply, including information on the calculation of standard errors, tests of significance for change over time, and use of the data for rural-urban analysis.

Chapter 1 – Understanding the supply, distribution, and educational pipeline of nurses is key to designing programs and policies that will ensure access to care and an effective health care system. This report analyzes data from a variety of sources to present recent trends and the current status of the registered nurse (RN) and licensed practical nurse (LPN) workforces.

Chapter 2 – This technical document is a companion to the report *The U.S. Nursing Workforce: Trends in Supply and Education.* It provides additional information on data and methodology for analysis of the nurse supply, including information on the calculation of standard errors, tests of significance for change over time, and use of the data for rural-urban analysis.

In: U.S. Nursing Workforce
Editor: Marla Parris

ISBN: 978-1-63463-540-0
© 2015 Nova Science Publishers, Inc.

Chapter 1

THE U.S. NURSING WORKFORCE: TRENDS IN SUPPLY AND EDUCATION[*]

National Center for Health Workforce Analysis

EXECUTIVE SUMMARY

Understanding the supply and distribution of nurses is key to ensuring access to care and an effective health care system. This report presents data on the supply, distribution, and education/pipeline of the U.S. nursing workforce. The data come from a variety of sources and present recent trends and the current status of the registered nurse (RN) and licensed practical/vocational (LPN) workforces. The report is intended to be used by national and state workforce planners, as well as educators, researchers, and policy makers.

The Current Supply of Nurses and Trends over Time[1]

- There were 2.8 million RNs (including advanced practice RNs) and 690,000 LPNs in the nursing workforce—that is, working in the field of nursing or seeking nursing employment in 2008 to 2010. About

---

[*] This is an edited, reformatted and augmented version of a report issued by the Health Resources and Services Administration, U.S. Department of Health and Human Services, October 2013.

- 445,000 RNs and 166,000 LPNs lived in rural areas (about 16 percent of the RN workforce and 24 percent of the LPN workforce).
- The nursing workforce grew substantially in the 2000s, with RNs growing by more than 500,000 (24.1 percent) and LPNs by more than 90,000 (15.5 percent).
- Growth in the nursing workforce outpaced growth in the U.S. population. The number of RNs per 100,000 population (per capita) increased by about 14 percent, and the number of LPNs per capita increased by about 6 percent.
- Owing to strong growth in new entrants, the absolute number of RNs younger than 30 has increased. Nevertheless, about one-third of the nursing workforce is older than 50. The average age of nurses has increased over the past decade, by almost two years for RNs and 1.75 years for LPNs, reflecting aging within the very large cohort of nurses aged 41 to 50 in 2000.
- Currently, about 55 percent of the RN workforce holds a bachelor's or higher degree. An associate's degree in nursing was the first nursing degree for many of these nurses. RNs are more likely to hold bachelor's or graduate degrees today than was true in 2000, but only by 5 percentage points.
- The RN and LPN workforces are slowly becoming more diverse over time. The proportion of non-white RNs and LPNs increased by about 5 percentage points during the past decade. The proportion of men in the RN workforce increased by about a percentage point and is currently 9 percent.
- The majority of RNs (63.2 percent) are providing inpatient and outpatient care in hospitals. The distribution of RNs across settings held relatively steady over the past decade. However, while the proportion of RNs in hospitals held steady, the number of RNs working in hospitals increased by more than 350,000 (about 25 percent). In contrast to RNs, less than one-third of LPNs (29.3 percent) work in hospitals, and that proportion has declined slightly over the past decade.

The RN and LPN Pipeline[2]

- The nursing pipeline, measured by the annual number of individuals who pass national nurse licensing exams, grew substantially from

2001 to 2011, with RN test passers growing 108 percent and LPN passers growing 80 percent. In 2011, more than 142,000 new graduate RNs passed the NCLEX-RN®. This compares with 68,561 in 2001.
- From 2001 to 2011, the number of bachelor's prepared RN candidates taking the NCLEXRN exam for the first time more than doubled, from 24,832 individuals in 2001 to 58,246 in 2011. Non-bachelor's prepared RN candidates taking the NCLEX-RN exam for the first time experienced a 96.5-percent growth, increasing from 43,927 in 2001 to 86,337 in 2011. Non-bachelor's prepared RN candidates continue to constitute the majority of all RN candidates (60 percent in 2011).
- The number of internationally educated RNs passing the NCLEX fluctuated significantly between 2001 and 2011. While not all enter the United States, passage of the NCLEX is a prerequisite and sets the maximum number of internationally educated RNs that can be licensed each year. From 2001 to 2007, the annual number of passers increased steadily, from about 6,700 to nearly 23,000. Perhaps as a result of the growing number of U.S. graduates and the recession, the annual number of internationally educated NCLEX passers has dropped since 2007 and was only 6,100 in 2011.

Post-Licensure Education[3]

- Nearly 28,000 RNs were awarded a post-licensure bachelor's degree in nursing (RN-BSN) in 2011. There has been an estimated 86.3-percent increase in the annual number of RNBSN graduates over just the past four years. This is important to achieve the higher level of education for RNs recommended by the Institute of Medicine for the vital role they play in the delivery of care in today's complex health care system.
- More than 24,000 nursing master's degrees and nearly 2,200 nursing doctoral degrees were awarded in 2011. The number of master's and doctoral graduates increased by 67 percent from 2007 to 2011.

This report on trends in the national nursing supply and pipeline does not take into account the many factors likely to influence future supply and demand. Therefore, the report does not address whether supply and demand will be in balance over the next decade.

The key indicators tracked in this report should be followed closely in the coming years as economic recovery, demographics, and health reform evolve to shape nursing workforce supply and demand in the United States.

INTRODUCTION

This report presents an overview of the trends in the supply and pipeline of nurses to assist the work of national and state officials, policy makers, the nursing community, educators, and researchers focused on the nursing workforce.

Data and information are incorporated from various sources covering both the registered nurse (RN) and licensed practical/vocational nurse (LPN) workforces. The sources vary in the years of data available, but where possible, trends over the past decade are analyzed.

Section 1, *The Registered Nurse and Licensed Practical/Vocational Nurse Workforce*, presents an overview and analysis of recent trends in the nurse supply.

This section includes estimates of RNs and LPNs working in each state, rural/urban differences, and trends in educational attainment, employment, and demographics of the nursing workforce such as age, race/ ethnicity and gender. Sources of data used for this section include the U.S. Census Bureau's American Community Survey 2008 to 2010 and the Census 2000 Long Form.

Section 2, *Nursing Pipeline and Education Capacity*, presents current information on the pipeline for nursing (the production of new nurses) nationally and by state. Data are also presented on the growth in newly licensed nurses, by degree type, the growth in internationally born/ educated nurses and trends in post-licensure education. The data used in this section were obtained from the National Council of State Boards of Nursing and the American Association of Colleges of Nursing.

SECTION 1. THE REGISTERED NURSE AND LICENSED PRACTICAL NURSE WORKFORCE

An analysis of recent trends in the nursing workforce is important to anticipate future supply growth and identify likely changes in educational and demographic composition.

Information on the size of the U.S. nursing workforce and its distribution across states and in rural and urban areas is presented. Growth in the workforce over time is measured against growth in the general population. Next, key trends in educational attainment, racial/ethnic composition, and gender are highlighted. The section concludes with an analysis of trends in the setting and work hours of the nursing workforce.

Two sources of data from the U.S. Census Bureau were used to examine the current supply of registered nurses (RNs) and licensed practical nurses (LPNs), as well as changes in the workforce that have occurred during the past decade: the American Community Survey (ACS) three-year combined file for 2008 to 2010 and the Census 2000 Long Form 5-percent sample. (See "About the Data" below.)

Owing to the household sampling strategy of these Census surveys, all results presented in this section are for the nursing *workforce*—those individuals who report their current occupation as nursing and who currently have or are seeking a job. It is not possible to count, with either data source, the number of individuals educated or licensed as nurses who are working in another field or are out of the workforce entirely.

Another important note is that advanced practice registered nurses are included in results for RNs. The Census data sources used here do not separate them.

About the Data

The ACS 2008 to 2010 three-year file and Census 2000 Long Form 5-percent sample offer nearly identical question wording and an established set of techniques for comparing results over time. The sources also offer large sample sizes: more than 110,000 RNs and 31,000 LPNs are included within the 2000 5-percent sample, while nearly 90,000 RNs and more than 21,000 LPNs are included in the ACS 2008 to 2010 three-year file. This means that estimates derived from these sources are highly precise and, in most cases, can be made at both state and national levels.

The ACS 2008 to 2010 three-year file was selected over a single-year file in order to improve the precision of state and national estimates. Unlike the Census 2000 data, which represent a point in time, the ACS three-year file represents an average of the three-year time period. It is inappropriate to refer to this estimate as representing 2009. Throughout this section, we refer to this as the "current" nurse supply because it was the most up-to-date three-year file available at the time of our analysis.

> For most estimates, relative standard errors (RSEs) are quite small. Because of the large sample size, even small differences across time (1 or 2 percentage points) are statistically significant at the 0.05 level. All differences over time discussed within the text of this section are statistically significant, though detailed results of significance testing are not presented.
>
> All estimates reported in this section have an RSE of less than 30 percent. More information about the data sources and methods used in this report can be found in "The U.S. Nursing Workforce: Technical Documentation," available at http://bhpr.hrsa.gov/healthworkforce/index.html.

Workforce Size and Distribution

There were an estimated 2,824,641 RNs and 690,038 LPNs within the nursing workforce during the 2008 to 2010 time period. Based on the size of the U.S. population during the period, this equates to 921 RNs and 225 LPNs per 100,000 members of the population (per capita). Tables 1 and 2, below, show the RN and LPN workforces by state, based on the ACS 2008 to 2010 three-year file.

Nurses who live in one state but work in another were placed according to the state in which they work. The total population in each state, also derived from the ACS three-year file, was used to calculate the number of RNs per 100,000 population in each state.

As Table 1 shows, the per capita supply of RNs varies substantially across states, from a high of 1,248 in South Dakota to a low of 678 in Idaho. Per capita RN supply does not take into account differences in population age, disease prevalence, or the number of hospital beds that must be staffed. Still, it is informative because it illustrates that national-level information masks substantial local-level differences. Figures 1 and 2 present the information graphically, showing that states located in the West and West South Central Census areas tend to have a lower per capita supply of RNs, whereas states in the Midwest and Northeast tend to have a higher per capita supply.

Table 2 and Figures 3 and 4 present the same information for LPNs. Similar to the density of RNs, LPN density is lowest in Western states. In general, areas of the country with a comparatively dense population of RNs also have a comparatively dense population of LPNs.

Table 1. The RN Workforce, by State, per 100,000 Population

State[1]	RNs	Total Population	RNs per 100,000
Alabama	45,666	4,753,812	960.6
Alaska	5,605	700,113	800.6
Arizona	50,841	6,345,751	801.2
Arkansas	27,415	2,897,671	946.1
California	274,722	36,971,641	743.1
Colorado	43,480	4,970,333	874.8
Connecticut	37,555	3,561,486	1,054.5
Delaware	10,380	891,791	1,163.9
District of Columbia[2]	9,869	592,306	1,666.2
Florida	167,476	18,674,425	896.8
Georgia	75,976	9,612,759	790.4
Hawaii	9,357	1,347,518	694.4
Idaho	10,527	1,553,404	677.7
Illinois	120,203	12,795,658	939.4
Indiana	63,655	6,458,253	985.6
Iowa	33,378	3,033,163	1,100.4

Table 1. (Continued)

State[1]	RNs	Total Population	RNs per 100,000
Kansas	28,556	2,833,318	1,007.9
Kentucky	44,755	4,317,738	1,036.5
Louisiana	42,856	4,490,487	954.4
Maine	16,153	1,329,222	1,215.2
Maryland	55,944	5,733,779	975.7
Massachusetts	80,725	6,514,611	1,239.1
Michigan	89,445	9,908,690	902.7
Minnesota	57,639	5,279,601	1,091.7
Mississippi	29,016	2,958,873	980.6
Missouri	63,756	5,960,413	1,069.7
Montana	11,172	983,763	1,135.6
Nebraska	22,260	1,813,164	1,227.7
Nevada	19,428	2,680,981	724.7
New Hampshire	13,860	1,316,255	1,053.0
New Jersey	75,269	8,756,104	859.6
New Mexico	15,701	2,037,799	770.5
New York	196,189	19,303,930	1,016.3
North Carolina	90,663	9,440,195	960.4
North Dakota	7,702	665,681	1,157.0
Ohio	126,582	11,526,823	1,098.2
Oklahoma	29,366	3,716,087	790.2
Oregon	32,113	3,805,432	843.9
Pennsylvania	140,077	12,662,926	1,106.2
Rhode Island	12,744	1,053,846	1,209.3
South Carolina	42,254	4,585,057	921.6

State[1]	RNs	Total Population	RNs per 100,000
South Dakota	10,076	807,563	1,247.7
Tennessee	67,159	6,303,437	1,065.4
Texas	186,573	24,789,312	752.6
Utah	18,771	2,720,974	689.9
Vermont	6,528	624,976	1,044.5
Virginia	64,268	7,928,022	810.6
Washington	56,607	6,658,052	850.2
West Virginia	19,220	1,847,352	1,040.4
Wisconsin	60,813	5,667,100	1,073.1
Wyoming	4,296	556,787	771.6
U.S. Total	2,824,641	306,738,434	920.9

Data Source: HRSA analysis of the ACS 2008-2010 three-year file
1 All state estimates have a relative standard error (RSE) of less than 10%.
2 The nursing workforce is likely denser in the District of Columbia (D.C.) in part because of the presence of several academic medical centers, like most cities, that require a large RN workforce. Many nurses and patients commute into D.C. for work and health services. Since most states include rural and/or suburban areas, it is not instructive to compare D.C. with states in terms of per capita supply.

Table 2. The LPN Workforce, by State, per 100,000 Population

State	LPNs	Total Population	LPNs per 100,000
Alabama	12,297	4,753,812	258.7
Alaska[3]	782	700,113	111.7
Arizona	7,853	6,345,751	123.8
Arkansas	10,734	2,897,671	370.4
California	54,817	36,971,641	148.3
Colorado	5,843	4,970,333	117.6
Connecticut	8,605	3,561,486	241.6
Delaware[2]	1,679	891,791	188.3
District of Columbia[1]	1,982	592,306	334.6

Table 2. (Continued)

State	LPNs	Total Population	LPNs per 100,000
Florida	45,686	18,674,425	244.6
Georgia	22,076	9,612,759	229.7
Hawaii[2]	2,107	1,347,518	156.4
Idaho[1]	2,880	1,553,404	185.4
Illinois	20,949	12,795,658	163.7
Indiana	17,114	6,458,253	265.0
Iowa	7,397	3,033,163	243.9
Kansas	7,056	2,833,318	249.0
Kentucky	9,857	4,317,738	228.3
Louisiana	17,457	4,490,487	388.8
Maine[1]	1,952	1,329,222	146.9
Maryland	11,733	5,733,779	204.6
Massachusetts	14,390	6,514,611	220.9
Michigan	19,196	9,908,690	193.7
Minnesota	15,462	5,279,601	292.9
Mississippi	9,719	2,958,873	328.5
Missouri	18,841	5,960,413	316.1
Montana[2]	1,737	983,763	176.6
Nebraska	5,882	1,813,164	324.4
Nevada	3,101	2,680,981	115.7
New Hampshire[1]	3,526	1,316,255	267.9
New Jersey	16,584	8,756,104	189.4
New Mexico[1]	2,555	2,037,799	125.4

State	LPNs	Total Population	LPNs per 100,000
New York	46,063	19,303,930	238.6
North Carolina	20,535	9,440,195	217.5
North Dakota[2]	2,802	665,681	420.9
Ohio	36,934	11,526,823	320.4
Oklahoma	13,335	3,716,087	358.8
Oregon[1]	2,998	3,805,432	78.8
Pennsylvania	38,202	12,662,926	301.7
Rhode Island[1]	1,735	1,053,846	164.6
South Carolina	10,149	4,585,057	221.3
South Dakota[2]	2,149	807,563	266.1
Tennessee	23,373	6,303,437	370.8
Texas	58,189	24,789,312	234.7
Utah[1]	2,728	2,720,974	100.3
Vermont[2]	1,229	624,976	196.6
Virginia	22,276	7,928,022	281.0
Washington	8,226	6,658,052	123.5
West Virginia	6,346	1,847,352	343.5
Wisconsin	10,279	5,667,100	181.4
Wyoming	641	556,787	115.1
U.S. Total	690,038	306,738,434	225.0

Data Source: HRSA analysis of the ACS 2008-2010 three-year file
Note: The LPN population in small states is more difficult to estimate with precision. Higher RSEs in these states mean less precise estimates.
[1]State has an RSE between 10% and 14.9%.
[2]State has an RSE between 15% and 19.9%.
[3]State has an RSE between 20% and 25%.

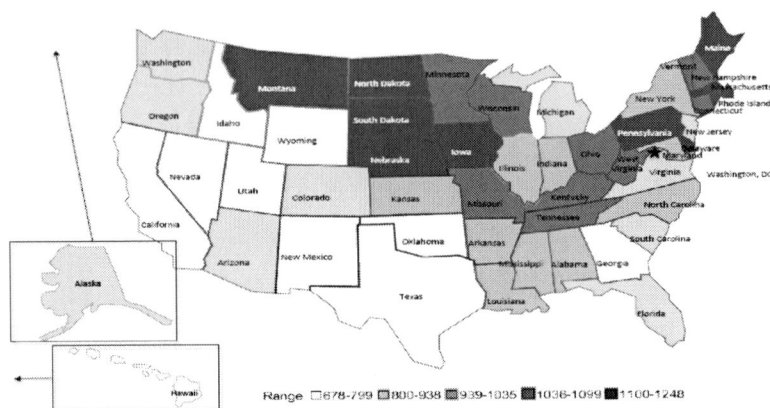

Data Source: HRSA analysis of the ACS 2008-2010 three-year file

Figure 1. The RN Workforce per 100,000 Population, by State.

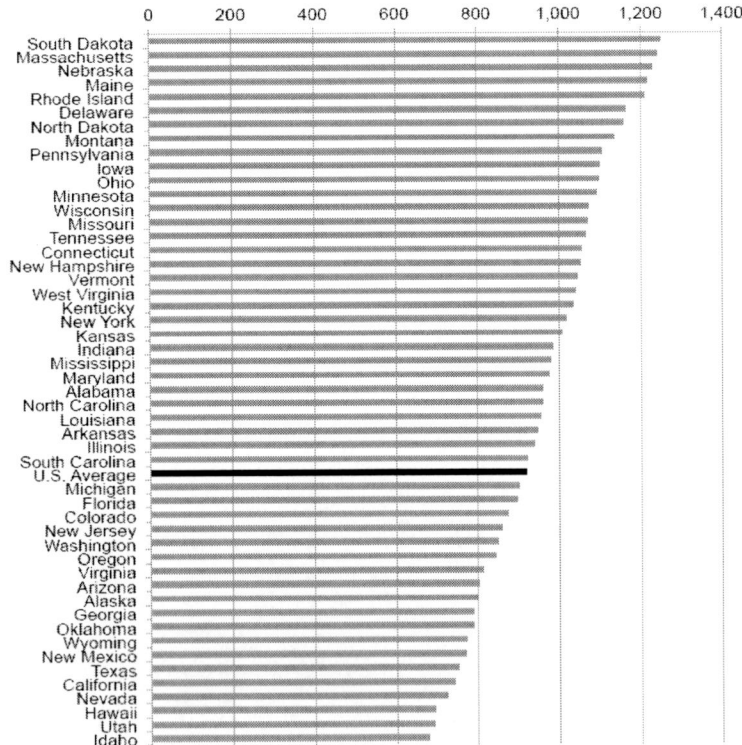

Data Source: HRSA analysis of the ACS 2008-2010 three-year file.

Figure 2. The per Capita RN Workforce, Ranked by State.

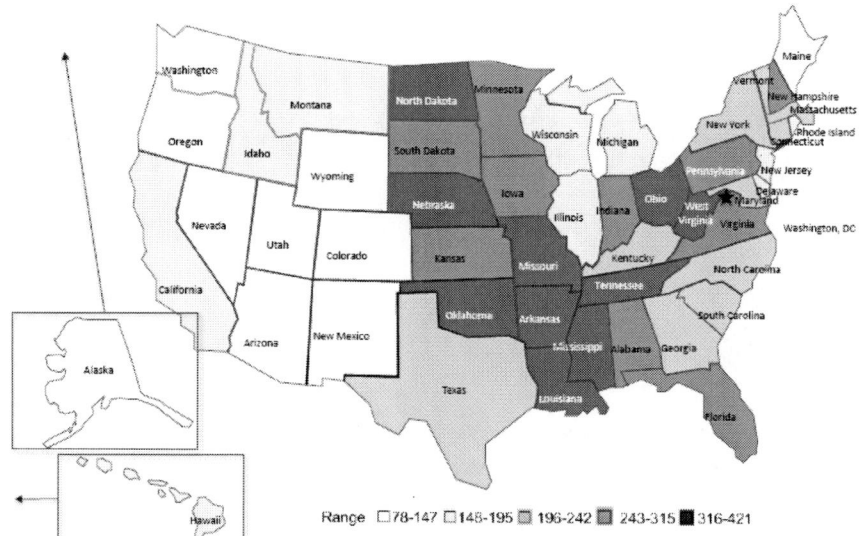

Data Source: HRSA analysis of the ACS 2008-2010 three-year file

Figure 3. The LPN Workforce per 100,000 Population, by State.

Workforce Distribution across Rural and Urban Areas

A large majority of nurses reside in urban areas, consistent with the distribution of the total population.[4] About 445,000 RNs and 166,000 LPNs reside in rural areas (see Figure 5). Almost one-quarter of LPNs (24 percent) live in rural areas, whereas only 16 percent of RNs do so. For comparison, about 17 percent of the U.S. population, or more than 52 million residents (as estimated in the ACS 2008 to 2010), live in rural areas.

Urban areas have a somewhat higher number of RNs per capita than is true for the nation as a whole, while rural areas have a lower per capita supply of RNs (see Figure 6). In contrast, rural areas have a higher number of LPNs per capita, compared with the nation, while urban areas have a lower per capita supply of LPNs.

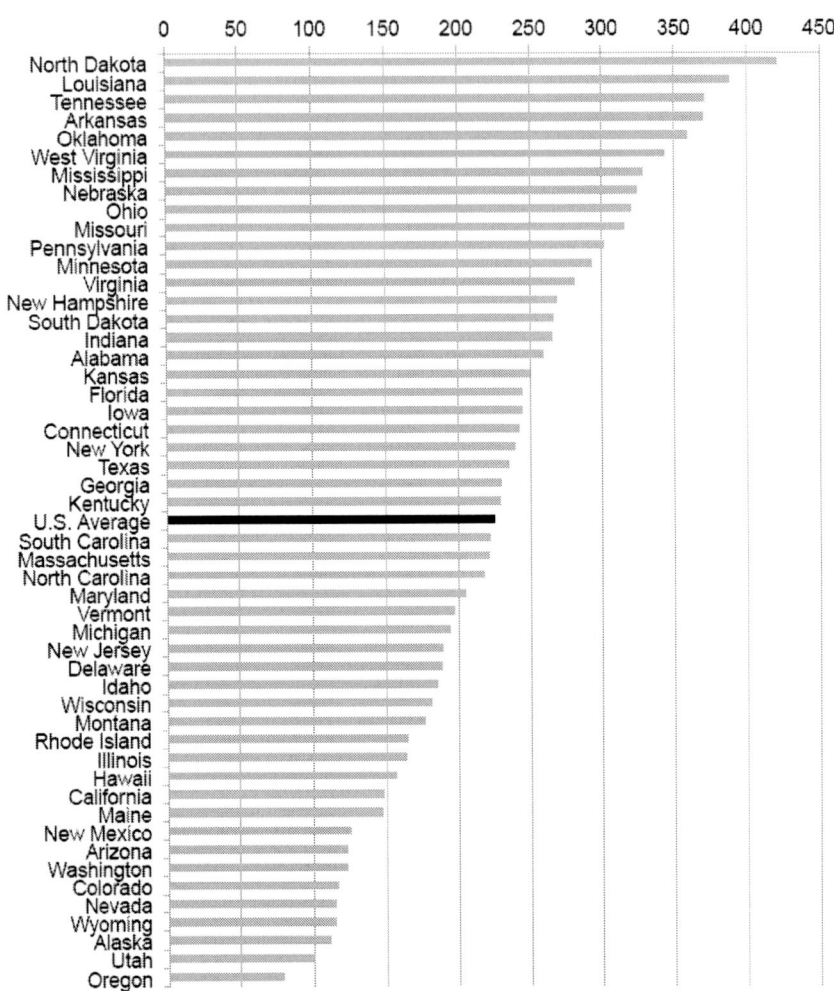

Data Source: HRSA analysis of the ACS 2008-2010 three-year file

Figure 4. The per Capita LPN Workforce, Ranked by State.

The U.S. Nursing Workforce: Trends in Supply and Education   15

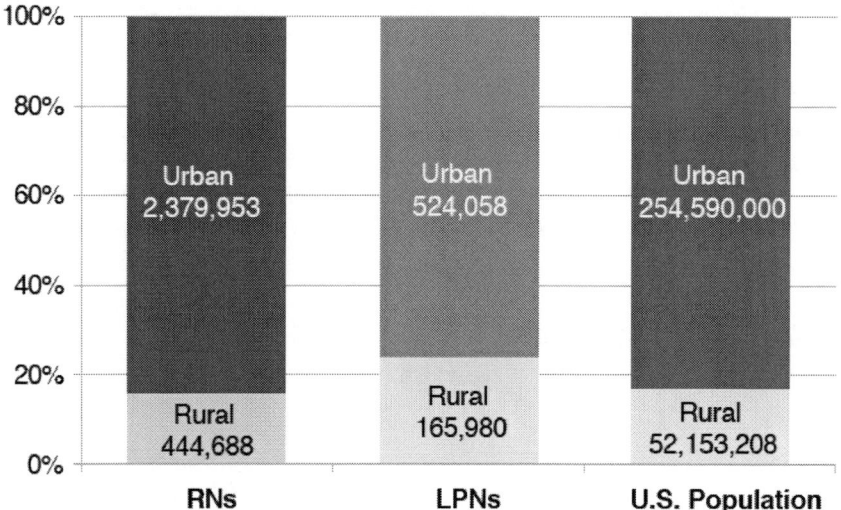

Data Source: HRSA analysis of the ACS 2008-2010 three-year file

Figure 5. Nursing Workforce Distribution in Rural and Urban Areas.

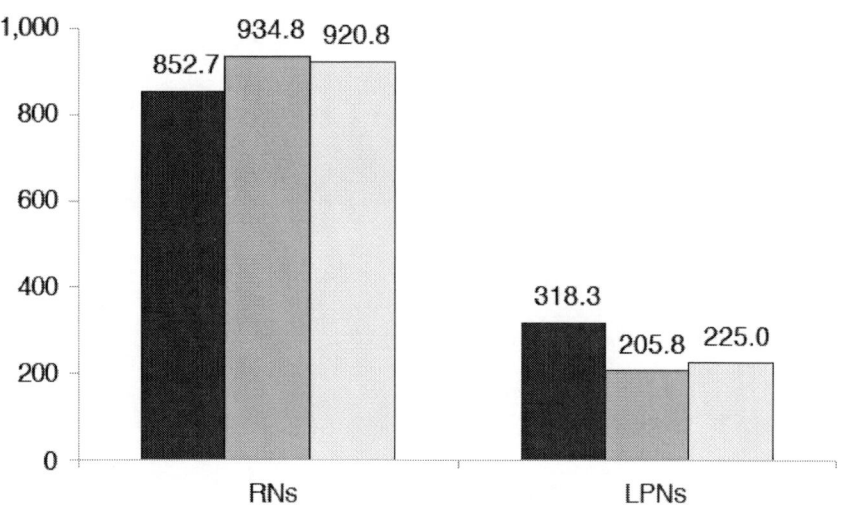

■ Per Capita Rural   ■ Per Capita Urban   □ Per Capita U.S.

Data Source: HRSA analysis of the ACS 2008-2010 three-year file.

Figure 6. Nurses per 100,000 Residents in Rural and Urban Areas.

Tables 3 and 4 present key demographic and employment characteristics for rural, urban, and all areas. In general, RNs in rural areas are more likely to be female and white non-Hispanic/ Latino and to hold an associate's degree or less as their highest degree. RNs in rural areas are slightly less likely to work in hospitals and more likely to work in nursing care facilities when compared with their urban counterparts. Similar demographic and setting differences were found among LPNs. Each of these characteristics is charted over time for the nation (rural and urban areas combined) in the next section.

Table 3. Residential Distribution of the RN Workforce Across Urban and Rural Areas

	Urban Areas (%)	Rural Areas (%)	All Areas (%)
Age			
25 or younger	5.3	4.9	5.2
26-30*	9.7	9.0	9.6
31-35	11.0	10.7	11.0
36-40	12.5	12.6	12.5
41-45	12.2	12.5	12.3
46-50	14.4	14.9	14.5
51-55	15.1	15.3	15.1
56-60*	11.2	11.9	11.3
61-65	5.9	5.7	5.9
66-70	1.8	1.7	1.8
71 or older	0.8	0.8	0.8
Total	100	100	100
Average Age	44.6	44.9	44.6
Education			
RN Diploma*	6.8	7.8	6.9
Associate's*	35.3	51.6	37.9
Bachelor's*	46.6	33.9	44.6
Master's and Doctoral*	11.4	6.8	10.6
Total	100	100	100
Race/Ethnicity			
White*	72.4	91.2	75.4
Black/African American*	10.9	4.3	9.9

	Urban Areas (%)	Rural Areas (%)	All Areas (%)
Hispanic/Latino*	5.4	1.8	4.8
Asian*	9.6	0.9	8.3
American Indian/Alaska Native*	0.7	0.3	0.4
Multiple/Other*	1.4	1.1	1.3
Total	100	100	100
Percent Male*	9.4	7.8	9.1
Setting			
Hospitals*	63.9	59.4	63.2
Nursing Care Facilities*	6.8	10.6	7.4
Offices of Physicians	4.8	4.5	4.8
Home Health Care Services*	3.6	4.6	3.8
Outpatient Care Centers*	4.5	5.3	4.6
Other Health Care Services*	5.6	4.6	5.4
Elementary and Secondary Schools	2.2	2.3	2.2
Employment Services	2.1	1.9	2.1
Insurance Carriers*	1.0	0.3	0.9
Administration of HR Programs[1]*	1.2	2.2	1.4
Justice, Public Order, and Safety[2]*	0.5	1.3	0.6
Offices of Other Practitioners*	0.3	0.2	0.3
Colleges and Universities*	0.6	0.4	0.6
Residential Facilities, w/o Nursing	0.3	0.5	0.4
All Other Settings[3]*	2.6	2.2	2.5
Total	100	100	100

Data Source: HRSA analysis of the ACS 2008-2010 three-year file
Note: Not all totals equal 100 due to rounding.
*Rural vs. urban proportions within the category are statistically significantly different at p<0.05.
[1] Category includes RNs whose jobs focus primarily on administration.
[2] Category includes the majority of nurses working in public health settings.
[3] For this analysis, all settings holding less than 1% of the RN population have been recoded to "Other."

Table 4. Residential Distribution of the LPN Workforce Across Urban and Rural Areas

	Urban Areas (%)	Rural Areas (%)	All Areas (%)
Age			
25 or younger	8.2	8.5	8.3
26-30	9.9	10.2	10.0
31-35	12.0	11.2	11.8
36-40	12.6	12.3	12.5
41-45	11.8	12.3	11.9
46-50	12.5	12.9	12.6
51-55	13.2	13.0	13.2
56-60	10.8	10.9	10.8
61-65	5.7	5.4	5.6
66-70	2.2	2.3	2.2
71 or older	1.1	1.3	1.2
Total	100	100	100
Average Age	43.6	43.6	43.6
Race/Ethnicity			
White*	56.9	83.2	63.2
Black/African American*	27.5	11.3	23.6
Hispanic/Latino*	8.9	3.2	7.5
Asian*	4.6	0.6	3.6
American Indian/Alaska Native	0.5	0.8	0.6
Multiple/Other*	1.6	1.0	1.4
Total	100	100	100
Percent Male*	8.5	4.8	7.6

	Urban Areas (%)	Rural Areas (%)	All Areas (%)
Age			
25 or younger	8.2	8.5	8.3
26-30	9.9	10.2	10.0
31-35	12.0	11.2	11.8
36-40	12.6	12.3	12.5
41-45	11.8	12.3	11.9
46-50	12.5	12.9	12.6
51-55	13.2	13.0	13.2
56-60	10.8	10.9	10.8
61-65	5.7	5.4	5.6
66-70	2.2	2.3	2.2
71 or older	1.1	1.3	1.2
Total	100	100	100
Average Age	43.6	43.6	43.6
Race/Ethnicity			
White*	56.9	83.2	63.2
Black/African American*	27.5	11.3	23.6
Hispanic/Latino*	8.9	3.2	7.5
Asian*	4.6	0.6	3.6
American Indian/Alaska Native	0.5	0.8	0.6
Multiple/Other*	1.6	1.0	1.4
Total	100	100	100
Percent Male*	8.5	4.8	7.6

Table 4. (Continued)

Setting	Urban Areas (%)	Rural Areas (%)	All Areas (%)
Hospitals*	29.5	28.8	29.3
Nursing Care Facilities	29.8	33.5	30.7
Offices of Physicians*	8.1	8.8	8.2
Home Health Care Services	6.2	6.9	6.3
Outpatient Care Centers*	5.6	6.0	5.7
Other Health Care Services	7.5	5.6	7.0
Elementary and Secondary Schools*	1.0	1.3	1.1
Employment Services	4.2	2.7	3.8
Administration of HR Programs[1]	0.9	1.0	0.9
Justice, Public Order, and Safety[2]	1.2	1.6	1.3
Residential Facilities, w/o Nursing*	1.4	1.0	1.3
All Other Settings[3]	4.8	2.8	4.3
Total	100	100	100

Data Source: HRSA analysis of the ACS 2008-2010 three-year file
Note: Not all totals equal 100 due to rounding.
*Rural vs. urban proportions within the category are statistically significantly different at p<0.05.
[1] Category includes RNs whose jobs focus primarily on administration.
[2] Category includes the majority of nurses working in public health settings.
[3] For this analysis, all settings holding less than 1% of the RN population have been recoded to "Other." Settings for which estimates had greater than 30% RSE have been recoded to "Other," including insurance carriers, colleges/universities, and offices of other health care practitioners.

Trends in the Nursing Workforce during the Past Decade

A comparison of estimates from the Census 2000 Long Form and the ACS 2008 to 2010 three-year file shows that the RN workforce grew by nearly one-quarter and the LPN workforce grew by 15.5 percent (see Figure 7). Over a period of approximately nine years, this equates to an annual growth of approximately 61,000 RNs (2.7-percent compound annual growth rate) and 10,300 LPNs (1.8-percent compound annual growth rate).

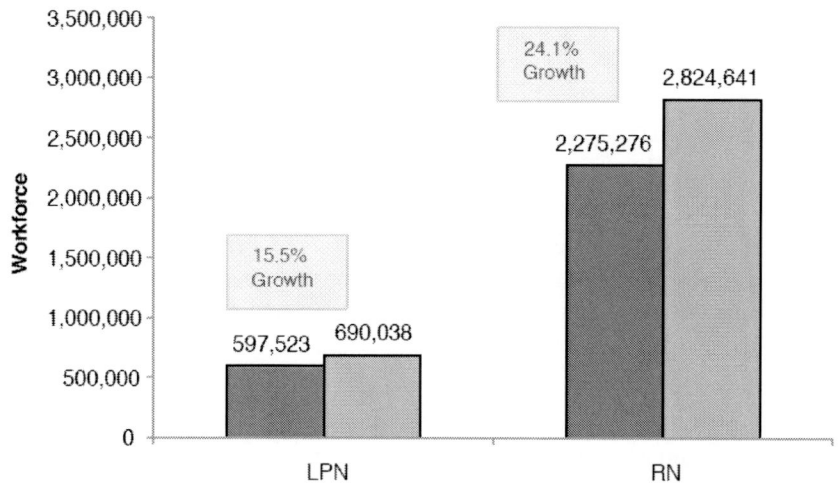

Data Sources: HRSA analysis of the ACS 2008-2010 three-year file and Census 2000 Long Form 5% sample

Figure 7. Growth in the U.S. Nursing Workforce.

Table 5. Growth in the per Capita Supply of RNs and LPNs

	Nurses (Census 2000)	Per Capita Supply (2000)	Nurses (ACS 08-10)	Per Capita Supply (08-10)	% Change in per Capita Supply
RNs	2,275,276	808.5	2,824,641	920.9	13.9%
LPNs	597,523	212.3	690,038	225.0	6.0%

Data Sources: HRSA analysis of the ACS 2008-2010 three-year file and Census 2000 Long Form 5% sample.

Over the past nine years, growth in the nursing workforce has surpassed that of the population. As Table 5 shows, the per capita supply of both RNs and LPNs has increased over time, with RN growth more than twice that for LPNs. The number of RNs per capita has increased by almost 14 percent, while the number of LPNs per capita has increased about 6 percent. Increasing per capita supply does not necessarily indicate that the nurse supply is more adequate now than it was in 2000. The measure does not account for other trends that have increased the demand for nurses, such as an aging population, increasing patient acuity, and hospital staffing and hiring preferences.

RN Workforce Education and Demographics

RNs can enter the workforce through education programs at multiple levels: diploma,[5] associate's, bachelor's, and even "entry" graduate degree programs that produce new nurses with master's degrees (see Figure 8). After entering the RN workforce, many nurses attain additional education to advance in their careers and to prepare them for advanced practice and teaching or research roles.

The Institute of Medicine (IOM) nursing report, entitled "Future of Nursing: Leading Change, Advancing Health," recommended higher levels of education in the nursing field. This recommendation was made to prepare nurses for the more complex care needed by sicker patients and the sophisticated new technologies available for providing care.[6] It was followed with a specific goal to increase the proportion of nurses with a bachelor's degree to 80 percent by 2020.

Analysis of Census data shows a small increase in the number of bachelor's and graduate degree holders—about 5 percentage points—over approximately nine years. Currently, about 55 percent of the RN workforce holds a bachelor's or higher degree. At this slow rate of change, it would take several decades to reach the 80-percent recommendation of the IOM. Rural areas have even further to go to meet the IOM recommendation: Only 34 percent of RNs in rural areas hold a bachelor's or higher degree (refer to Table 3). Section 2 presents information on both pre- and post-licensure bachelor's graduates.

The Age Structure of the RN Workforce

A key concern for workforce planners is the age distribution of the workforce, as an aging workforce portends large numbers of retirements. Over the past decade, the average age of RNs has increased by nearly two years, from 42.7 years in 2000 to 44.6 years in the ACS 2008 to 2010. Figure 9 provides a graphical view of the changing age structure of RNs over time. In 2000, a large proportion of RNs were 41 to 45 years old. In the ACS 2008 to 2010, the age distribution is flatter, and a larger proportion is older than age

50. Similar proportions fall into the younger age categories in both time periods, however.

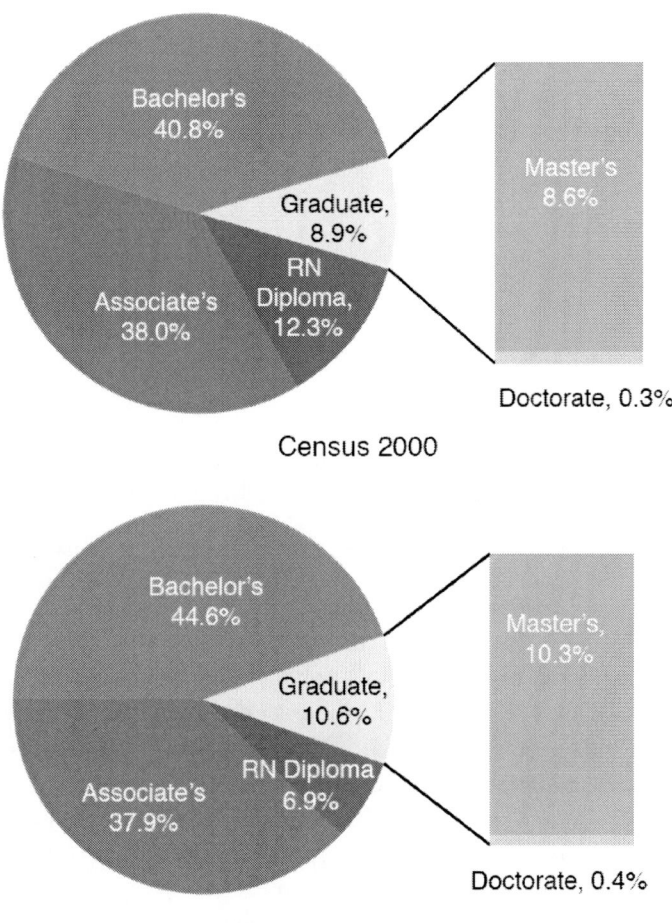

Census 2000

ACS 08-10

Data Sources: HRSA analysis of the ACS 2008-2010 three-year file and Census 2000 Long Form 5% sample

Figure 8. Highest Degree Held by RNs, Census 2000 and ACS 2008 to 2010.

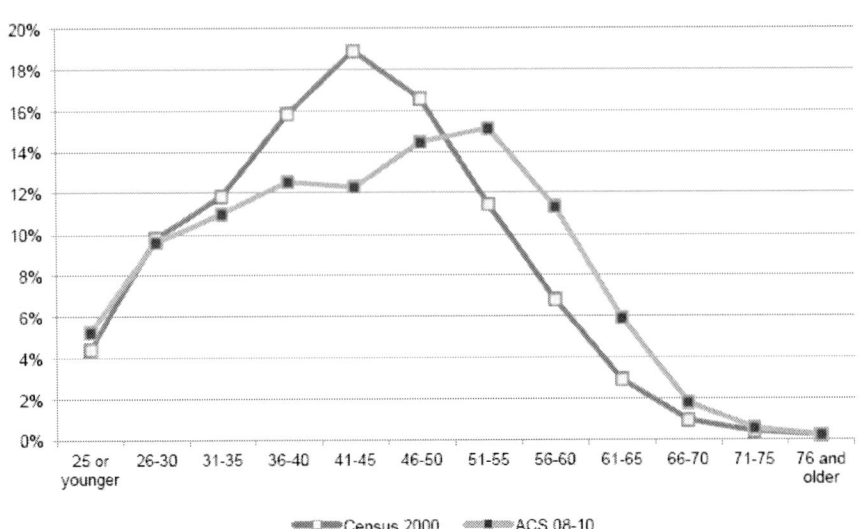

Data Sources: HRSA analysis of the ACS 2008-2010 three-year file and Census 2000 Long Form 5% sample.

Figure 9. The Changing Age Distribution of RNs, in Five-Year Increments.

Another way to view the changing age structure of nurses is through a comparison of absolute numbers in the workforce (see Figure 10). The workforce has grown overall, but this growth is concentrated in the older and younger ends of the age spectrum, and there are actually fewer RNs aged 36 to 45 working today, compared with nine years ago. Although the nursing workforce has aged over the past decade, it is encouraging to see growth in the number aged 35 and younger. This finding suggests that young people continue to see nursing as a viable career and predicts longer-term stability in the age distribution of the nursing workforce.

However, the tremendous growth of RN cohorts nearing retirement age is still a cause for concern. Over the next 10 to 15 years, the nearly 1 million RNs older than 50—about one-third of the current workforce—will reach retirement age. Retirement of large numbers of RNs over the next two decades means a loss of experiential knowledge and leadership brought to the workforce by seasoned RNs. Depending on the retirement decisions of this older cohort, which may be influenced by the pace of economic recovery, sudden spikes in retirement may exacerbate geographic and facility-level nursing shortages.

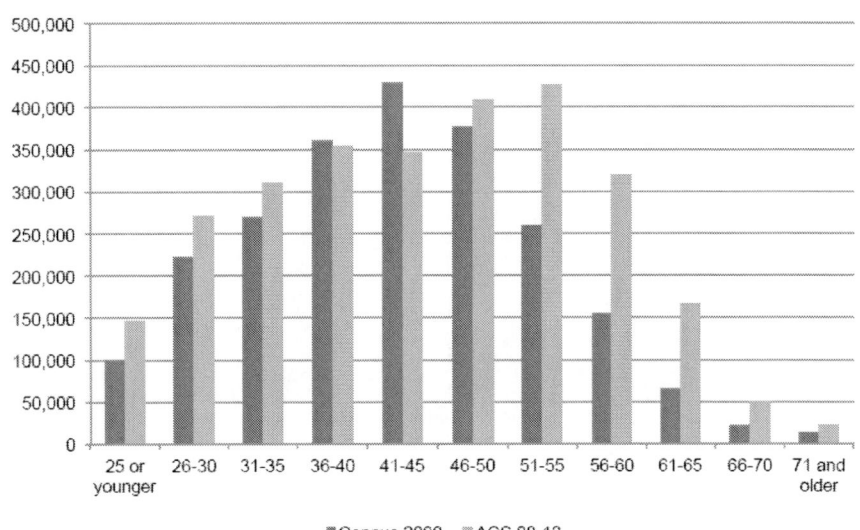

■ Census 2000   ■ ACS 08-10

Data Sources: HRSA analysis of the ACS 2008-2010 three-year file and Census 2000 Long Form 5% sample

Figure 10. Counts of RNs in the Workforce, by Age, in Five-Year Increments.

At the same time, health care delivery settings will need to accommodate an older nursing workforce over the next decade. As recommended by the Robert Wood Johnson Foundation in its 2006 white paper, *Wisdom at Work*,[7] employers will need to consider creative options for retaining older nurses. Such options include more flexible scheduling and new roles that take advantage of the older nurse's experience.

RN Workforce Diversity

Diversity within the nursing workforce—in terms of race/ethnicity and sex—is desirable because it can improve both access and care quality for minorities and medically underserved populations.[8] Nursing has historically been dominated by white females, and as Figure 11 shows, the nursing workforce is still predominantly white. However, over time, the proportion of racial/ethnic minorities has been increasing. Black/African Americans, Asians, and Hispanics/Latinos[9] make up greater proportions of the RN population, while whites have declined in proportion, from more than 80 percent in 2000 to about 75 percent in the ACS 2008 to 2010.

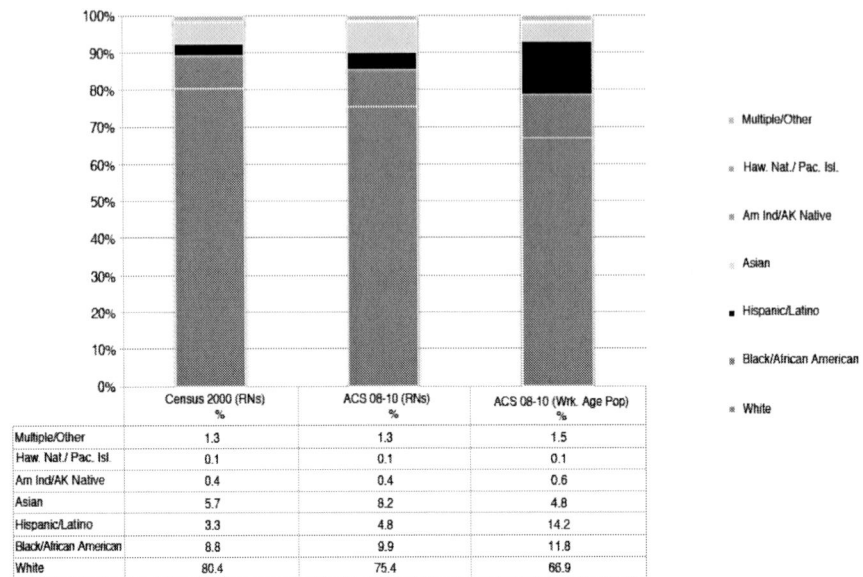

Data Sources: HRSA analysis of the ACS 2008-2010 three-year file and Census 2000 Long Form 5% sample

Figure 11. Race/Ethnicity in the RN Workforce and Total Working-Age Population.

Figure 11 also shows a comparison with the current U.S. working-age population (i.e., the population aged 16 and older) for race/ethnicity. The working-age population has a lower percentage of whites (67 percent vs. 75 percent for RNs). The RN workforce has a smaller percentage of Hispanics/Latinos and Black/African Americans, and a larger percentage of Asians, when compared with the total working-age population. The percentage difference for Hispanics/Latinos is particularly notable: They compose 14 percent of the working-age population but only 5 percent of the RN workforce.

Nursing remains a predominantly female profession, but the proportion of RNs who are male has increased over time: from 7.7 percent in Census 2000 to 9.1 percent in the ACS 2008 to 2010.

LPN Workforce Demographics

Many of the demographic trends observed for RNs hold for LPNs as well. As Figure 12 shows, the LPN age distribution has also flattened and shifted toward older ages. Also consistent with the findings for RNs, the proportion of younger nurses appears to be holding reasonably steady. During the time period covered by this analysis, the average age of LPNs increased by about 1.75 years, from 41.9 in 2000 to 43.6 in the ACS 2008 to 2010.

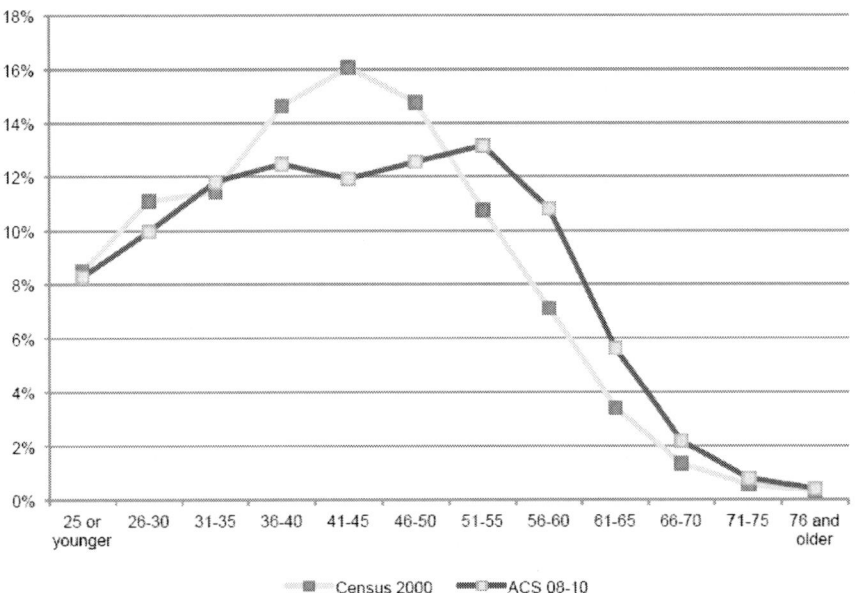

Data Sources: HRSA analysis of the ACS 2008-2010 three-year file and Census 2000 Long Form 5% sample.

Figure 12. Changing Age Distribution of LPNs, in Five-Year Increments.

Similar to RNs, the absolute number of LPNs has grown overall, but this growth has occurred only among those younger than 30 and older than 50 (see Figure 13). The number of LPNs aged 31 to 50 has actually decreased over the past 10 years. More than one-third of the LPN workforce is older than age 50.

The proportion of LPNs from minority racial/ethnic groups has increased over time (from about 32 percent to 37 percent), while the proportion reporting white race has declined (see Figure 14). LPNs are more likely to identify as racial/ethnic minorities when compared with RNs. In particular, the proportion of Black/African Americans is higher among LPNs (23.6 percent in the ACS 2008 to 2010 vs. 9.9 percent for RNs). As Figure 14 shows, the LPN workforce has a substantially higher percentage of African Americans than does the total working-age population. However, as was true for RNs, Hispanics/Latinos are notably underrepresented in the LPN workforce.

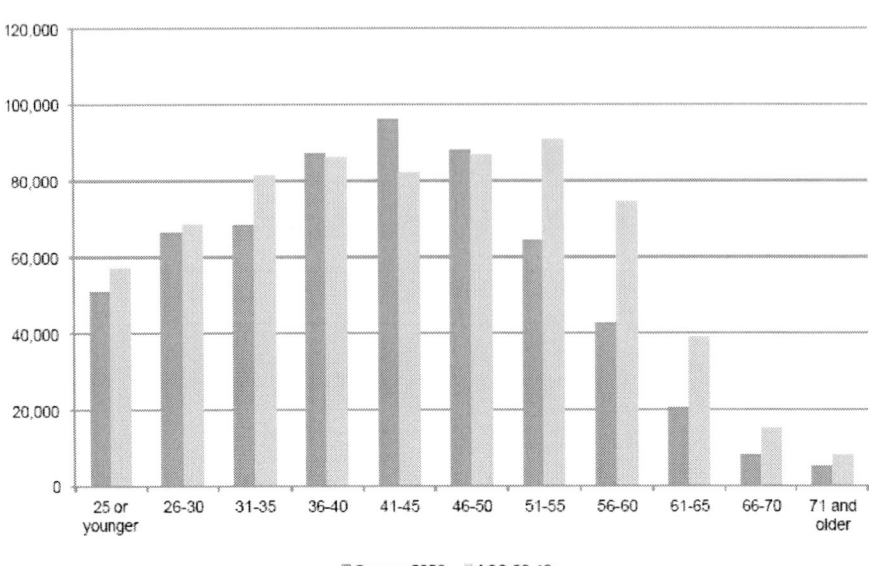

Data Sources: HRSA analysis of the ACS 2008-2010 three-year file and Census 2000 Long Form 5% sample.

Figure 13. Counts of LPNs in the Workforce, by Age, in Five-Year Increments.

Employment Characteristics of RNs and LPNs

The settings[10] in which nurses are employed are shown in Table 6. The majority of RNs (63.2 percent) continue to work in hospitals, and that proportion has not changed significantly during the past decade. Over time, the proportion working in nursing care facilities, physician offices, and home health has declined slightly, while the proportion working in outpatient care centers and "other health care services" has increased slightly. Note that these increases and decreases are quite small and that the majority of RNs are still providing inpatient and outpatient care in hospitals.

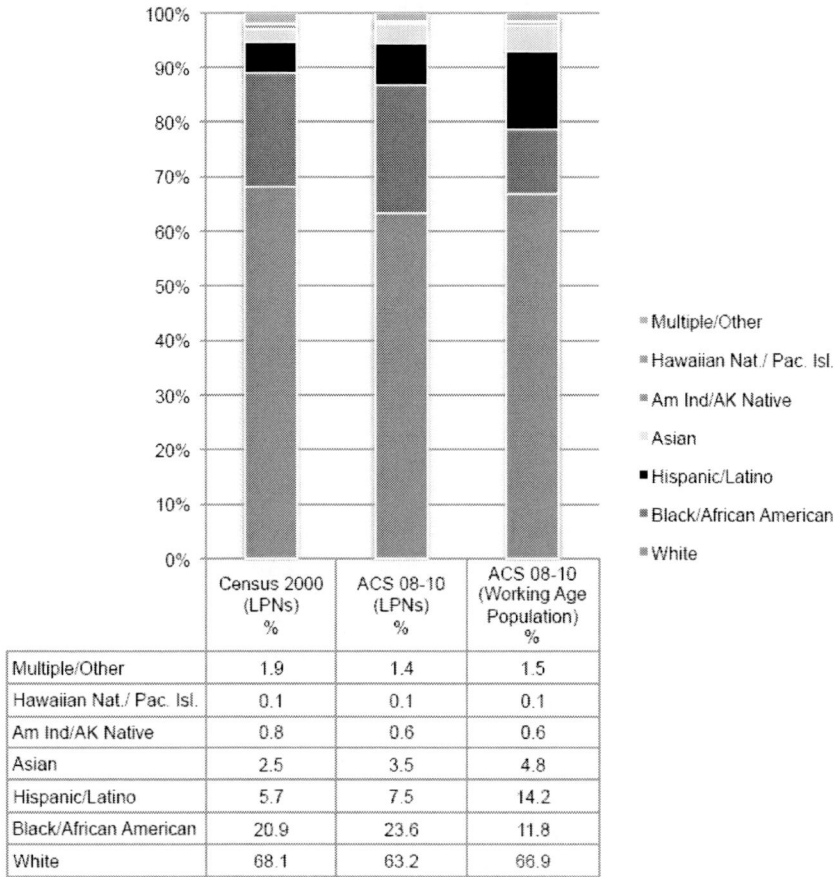

Data Sources: HRSA analysis of the ACS 2008-2010 three-year file and Census 2000 Long Form 5% sample

Figure 14. Race/Ethnicity in the LPN Workforce and Total Working-Age Population.

In sharp contrast, less than one-third of LPNs (29.3 percent) work in hospitals. That proportion has declined slightly (from 34.9 percent) during the past decade. Care provided by LPNs has shifted away from hospitals and physician offices and toward home health, outpatient care centers, and "other health care services." About one-third of LPNs work in nursing care facilities, and that proportion has held steady over time. LPNs compose the predominant licensed workforce within residential long-term care facilities.

Table 6. Setting of Employment for Nurses, Census 2000 and ACS 2008 to 2010

	RNs		LPNs	
	Census 2000 %	ACS 08-10 %	Census 2000 %	ACS 08-10 %
Hospitals	62.7	63.2	34.9	29.3
Nursing Care Facilities[1]	8.3	7.4	30.2	30.7
Offices of Physicians	6.9	4.8	11.2	8.2
Home Health Care Services	4.5	3.8	5.6	6.3
Outpatient Care Centers	3.1	4.6	3.6	5.7
Other Health Care Services	2.9	5.4	2.3	7.0
Elementary and Secondary Schools	2.3	2.2	0.8	1.7
Employment Services	2.0	2.1	3.4	3.8
Insurance Carriers and Related Activities	1.0	0.9	0.3	0.2
Administration of Human Resource Programs[2]	0.9	1.4	0.3	0.9
Justice, Public Order, and Safety Activities[3]	0.7	0.6	1.0	1.3
Offices of Other Health Practitioners	0.6	0.3	0.9	0.4
Colleges and Universities, Including Junior Colleges	0.6	0.6	0.2	0.3
Residential Care Facilities, Without Nursing	0.5	0.4	1.8	1.3
All Other Settings[4]	3.1	2.5	3.6	3.4

Data Sources: HRSA analysis of the ACS 2008-2010 three-year file and Census 2000 Long Form 5% sample

[1] Category includes skilled nursing facilities, also called nursing homes.
[2] Category includes RNs whose jobs focus primarily on administration.
[3] Category includes the majority of nurses working in public health settings.
[4] For this analysis, all settings holding less than 1% of the RN population have been recoded to "Other."

An alternative view is the growth or decline in the estimated number of workers, by setting, as shown for RNs in Table 7. The RN workforce grew by 24 percent during the decade, and most settings experienced increases in their RN workforces.

Even though the *percentage* of RNs working in hospitals did not increase significantly, the absolute *number* of RNs working in hospitals increased by more than 350,000—about 25 percent. Despite the growth in the RN workforce overall, three settings experienced absolute losses in RN employees: offices of physicians, offices of other health practitioners, and residential care facilities.[11]

The largest gains, as a percentage of growth in absolute numbers, occurred for outpatient care centers, administration positions, and "other healthcare services."

The LPN workforce grew by 15.5 percent over the past decade, but the growth was very uneven across settings (see Table 8). The number of LPNs in hospitals actually decreased by about 6,500, and the LPN workforce in the offices of physicians and other providers decreased by 12,000 during the past decade.

Large gains in absolute numbers occurred for nursing care facilities (31,366), outpatient care centers (17,921), home health (10,374), and "other health care services" (34,918).

The average number of hours worked by RNs held remarkably steady over the time period covered by this analysis, hovering at about 37 hours per week. When examined by age (see Figure 15), it is clear that older nurses are, as expected, working fewer hours than younger nurses. Interestingly, nurses aged 60 and older are working *more* hours in the ACS 2008 to 2010 when compared with Census 2000.

This finding may be due to the recession, which anecdotal reports suggest has increased the amount of time nurses work, owing to spouses who have suffered job losses and reductions in hours. It is unclear why the differences are found primarily among those older than 60, although the impact of the recession on retirement savings differentially impacts those who are closer to retirement.

Table 7. Estimated Number of RNs, by Setting of Employment

	Census 2000 Estimate	ACS 08-10 Estimate	Estimated Growth/Decline	% Change in Growth
Hospitals	1,427,497	1,785,304	357,807	25.1%
Nursing Care Facilities	189,594	208,051	18,457	9.7%
Offices of Physicians	156,559	134,231	-22,328	-14.3%
Home Health Care Services	101,895	105,922	4,027	4.0%
Outpatient Care Centers	70,224	131,022	60,798	86.6%
Other Health Care Services	66,723	153,449	86,726	130.0%
Elementary and Secondary Schools	51,495	61,323	9,828	19.1%
Employment Services	45,835	58,362	12,527	27.3%
Insurance Carriers and Related Activities	22,919	25,155	2,236	9.8%
Administration of Human Resource Programs[1]	20,509	38,136	17,627	85.9%
Justice, Public Order, and Safety Activities[2]	14,793	18,137	3,344	22.6%
Offices of Other Health Practitioners	13,346	7,596	-5,750	-43.1%
Colleges and Universities, Including Junior Colleges	12,637	16,320	3,683	29.1%
Residential Care Facilities, Without Nursing	10,853	9,928	-925	-8.5%
All Other Settings[3]	70,397	71,705	1,308	1.9%
Totals	2,275,276	2,824,641	549,365	24.1%

Data Sources: HRSA analysis of the ACS 2008-2010 three-year file and Census 2000 Long Form 5% sample

[1] Category includes RNs whose jobs focus primarily on administration.
[2] Category includes the majority of nurses working in public health settings.
[3] For this analysis, all settings holding less than 1% of the RN population have been recoded to "Other."

Table 8. Estimated Number of LPNs, by Setting of Employment

	Census 2000 Estimate	ACS 08-10 Estimate	Change Over Time	% Change in Estimates
Hospitals	208,757	202,247	-6,510	-3.1%
Nursing Care Facilities	180,228	211,594	31,366	17.4%
Offices of Physicians	66,915	56,874	-10,041	-15.0%
Home Health Care Services	33,225	43,599	10,374	31.2%
Outpatient Care Centers	21,613	39,534	17,921	82.9%
Other Health Care Services	13,612	48,530	34,918	256.5%
Elementary and Secondary Schools	4,907	7,312	2,405	49.0%
Employment Services	20,226	26,530	6,304	31.2%
Insurance Carriers and Related Activities	1,467	1,646	179	12.2%
Administration of Human Resource Programs[1]	2,039	6,426	4,387	215.2%
Justice, Public Order, and Safety Activities[2]	6,113	8,956	2,843	46.5%
Offices of Other Health Practitioners	5,084	2,565	-2,519	-49.5%
Colleges and Universities, Including Junior Colleges	1,255	2,291	1,036	82.5%
Residential Care Facilities, Without Nursing	10,715	8,721	-1,994	-18.6%
All Other Settings[3]	21,367	23,213	1,846	8.6%
Totals	597,523	690,038	92,515	15.5%

Data Sources: HRSA analysis of the ACS 2008-2010 three-year file and Census 2000 Long Form 5% sample

[1] Category includes RNs whose jobs focus primarily on administration.
[2] Category includes the majority of nurses working in public health settings.
[3] For this analysis, all settings holding less than 1% of the LPN population have been recoded to "Other."

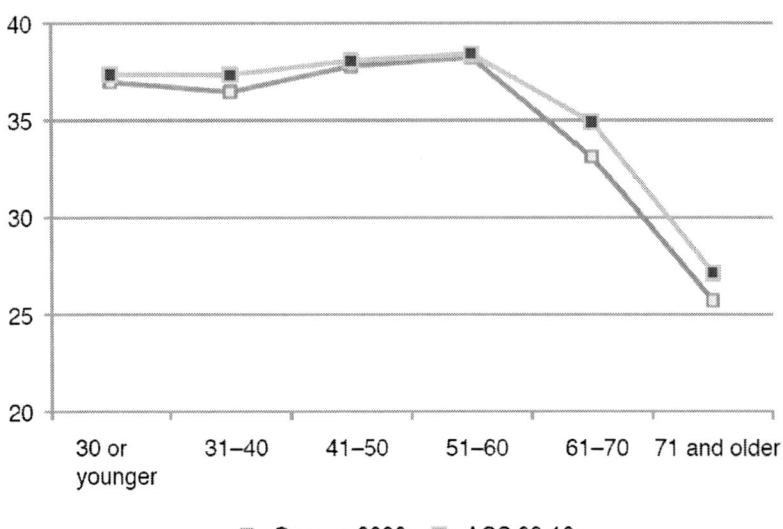

Data Sources: HRSA analysis of the ACS 2008-2010 three-year file and Census 2000 Long Form 5% sample.

Figure 15. Average Hours Worked by RNs, by Age.

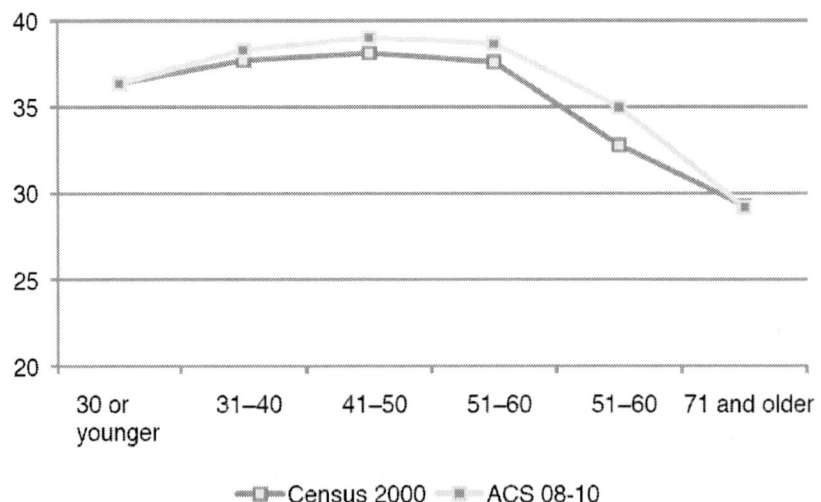

Data Sources: HRSA analysis of the ACS 2008-2010 three-year file and Census 2000 Long Form 5% sample.

Figure 16. Average Hours Worked by LPNs, by Age.

The average hours worked by LPNs also held quite steady over time, hovering around 37 hours per week across all ages. Similar to RNs, the ACS 2008 to 2010 data suggest that LPNs are working more hours than in 2000 within older age categories (refer to Figure 16). The difference is particularly noticeable in the 61 to 70 age category.

Figure 17 shows the average salary of a full-time nurse (36 or more hours per week). Full-time salary has increased by about $20,000 for RNs and about $11,500 for LPNs over the past decade. An increasing average salary can reflect the influence of many factors, including inflation, an older (and more experienced) workforce, and wage hikes to stimulate employment interest in areas facing a nursing shortage. Figure 17 presents the average salary within the ACS 2008 to 2010 adjusted to 2000 constant dollars to remove the impact of inflation (darker part of the bar). As the figure also shows, once inflation has been accounted for, the salary increase remains notable at nearly 15 percent ($6,600) over 10 years.

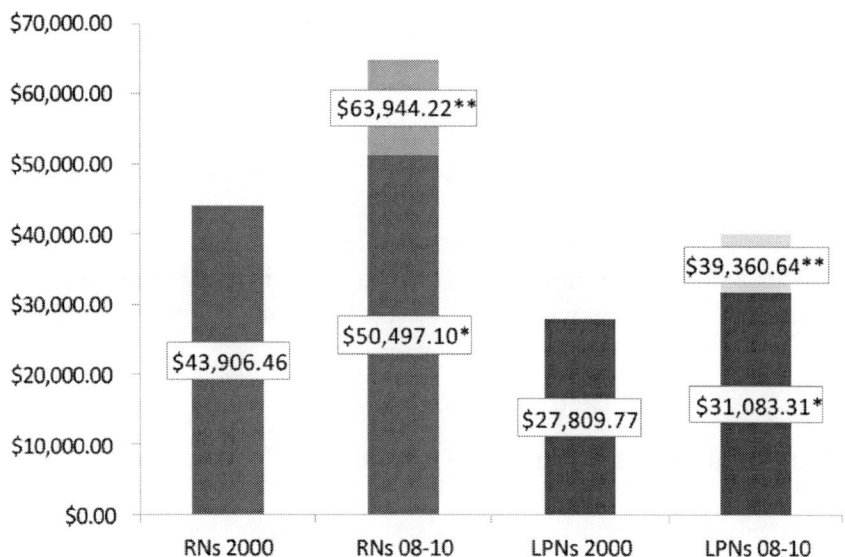

Data Sources: HRSA analysis of the ACS 2008-2010 three-year file and Census 2000 Long Form 5% sample
* Inflation adjusted to 2000 constant dollars.
**Actual salary in the ACS 2008-2010, adjusted to 2010 dollars.

Figure 17. Growth in Full-Time Nurse Salaries.

Section 2. Nursing Pipeline and Nursing Education Capacity

A key driver of the nurse supply in the future is the nation's capacity to produce new nurses through our education system—the workforce pipeline. In general, the pipeline can be viewed through a number of metrics, including the number of future students, current students, new graduates, or new licensees. However, measuring the nursing pipeline presents a particular analytic challenge for two reasons. First, new RNs enter the field from a variety of educational levels, including diploma, associate's, bachelor's, and master's degree programs. Second, many graduates of diploma and associate's degree programs return to school to earn higher degrees; thus, reports of bachelor's degree graduates often include both those entering nursing for the first time as well as RNs seeking the additional degree qualification. Similarly, while the vast majority of new master's degrees represent continuing education for existing nurses, some earning master's degrees are new nurses. As a result, it can be difficult to separate new nurses from existing nurses in data reported on the pool of nursing graduates.

Though there are different types of degrees awarded to those entering nursing, every individual who wishes to practice as a nurse in the United States must pass a licensure examination: the National Council Licensure Examination for Registered Nurses (NCLEX-RN®) or the National Council Licensure Examination for Practical Nurses (NCLEX-PN®).

This section of the report presents data on the two major components of the nursing workforce pipeline: new entrants to the profession and post-licensure education.

New Entrants to the Nursing Profession

Trends in U.S.-educated candidates both sitting for and passing the licensure exams are presented in Figures 18 through 23.

> **About the Data**
>
> Data for NCLEX exams are published annually to provide descriptive information, including pass rates by quarter, for licensure candidates by country of education (U.S. or international). Summary charts and tables in this section focus on U.S.-educated NCLEX exam passers.
>
> Additional data, including the jurisdiction of the test taker and educational attainment of NCLEX-RN candidates, are available only for first-time, U.S.-educated test takers. Therefore, this section also includes tables and figures that incorporate first-time test taker data where appropriate.
>
> First-time and repeat U.S.-educated candidates for the NCLEX-RN have pass rates of 87.4 percent and 54.9 percent, respectively. First- time and repeat U.S.-educated candidates for the NCLEX-PN have pass rates of 87.1 percent and 40.6 percent, respectively.
>
> Source: The National Council of State Boards of Nursing, Nurse Licensure and NCLEX Examination Statistics Publications, 20022012, Volumes 4, 13, 19, 20, 25, 31, 35, 42, 50, and 52, available at https://www.ncsbn.org/1236.htm.

Registered Nurses

Resulting from concerns about nurse shortages and calls to increase enrollment, the number of individuals pursuing nursing education has increased. Consequently, the number of nurses passing the exam required to become licensed as a nurse more than doubled between 2001 and 2011. As Figure 18 shows, the number of individuals passing the NCLEX-RN increased steadily over the course of the past 10 years, with particularly large increases in the middle of the decade. Though growth slowed somewhat from 2008 on, NCLEX volumes showed yearon-year increases even throughout the recent economic downturn.

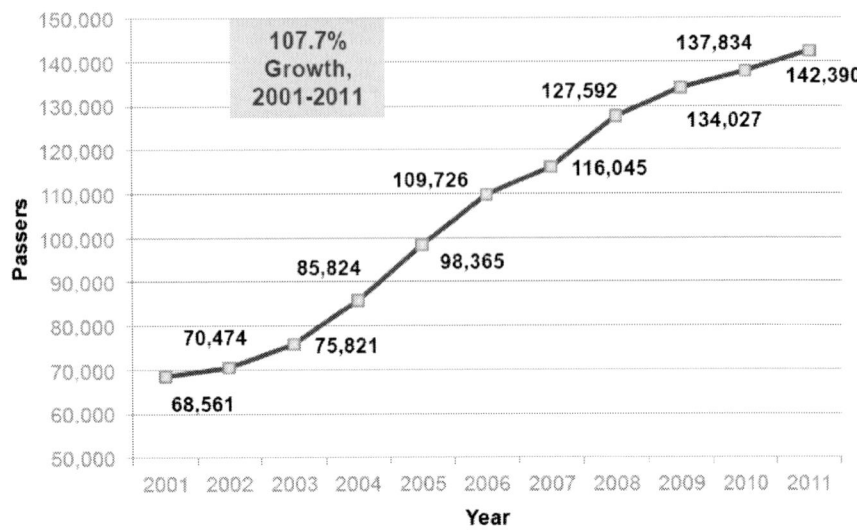

Data Source: HRSA compilation of data from the National Council of State Boards of Nursing, Nurse Licensure and NCLEX Examination Statistics Publications, 2002-2012, and from the National Council of State Boards of Nursing, "Number of Candidates Taking the NCLEX Examination and Percent Passing, by Type of Candidate," https://www.ncsbn.org/Table of Pass Rates 2011.pdf.

Figure 18. NCLEX-RN Passers, 2001 to 2011.

While data on overall growth in the nursing pipeline are critical to help inform projections of the size of the future workforce, NCLEX data can also provide more detailed information about licensure candidates to shed light on other key issues. A particular focus in the United States in recent years has been on the educational attainment of new nurses.

Figure 19 depicts the growth in first-time, U.S.-educated exam candidates by bachelor's and non-bachelor's degree status from 2001 to 2011. Bachelor's prepared candidates more than doubled, increasing by nearly 135 percent. Of the 75,824 additional individuals who sat for the NCLEX-RN in 2011, compared with 2001, 33,414 had obtained a bachelor's degree in nursing (BSN). Thus, bachelor's prepared candidates represented about 44 percent of the overall growth exhibited from 2001 to 2011.

Non-bachelor's test takers, a group consisting of diploma, associate's degree, and special program code NCLEX-RN candidates, grew by over 96 percent, from 43,927 in 2001 to 86,337 in 2011.

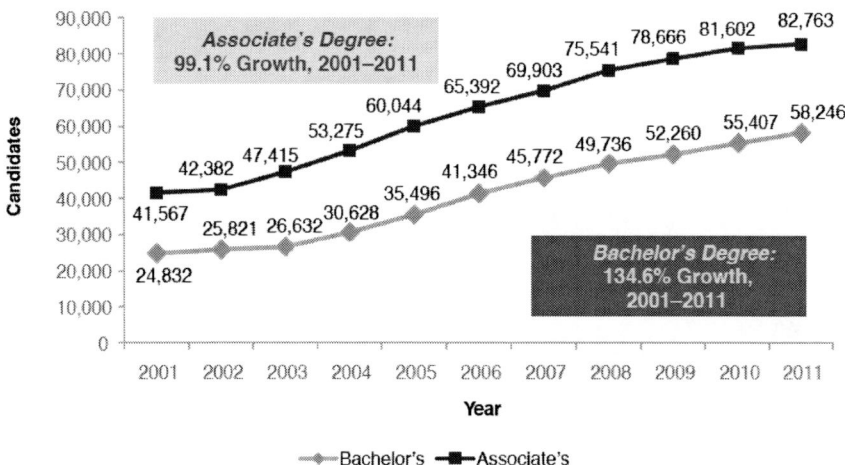

Data Source: HRSA compilation of data from the National Council of State Boards of Nursing, Nurse Licensure and NCLEX Examination Statistics Publications, 2002-2012, and from the National Council of State Boards of Nursing, "Number of Candidates Taking the NCLEX Examination and Percent Passing, by Type of Candidate," https://www.ncsbn.org/Table_of_Pass_Rates_2011.pdf.

Figure 19. Growth in NCLEX-RN First-Time Test Takers, by Bachelor's and Non-Bachelor's Degree Status, 2001 to 2011.

The faster growth of bachelor's prepared candidates over the course of the past decade caused the overall distribution of RN licensure test takers to shift slightly toward bachelor's prepared candidates. These candidates increased from 36.1 percent of the licensure pipeline in 2001 to just over 40 percent in 2011 (see Figure 20). Despite this shift, the majority of first-time candidates for RN licenses have not obtained a bachelor's degree. Of NCLEX-RN testers, 59.7 percent are not bachelor's prepared, and the vast majority of these individuals (95.8 percent) are educated at the associate's degree level.

Although the majority of examinees in 2011 continued to be educated at the associate's degree level, trends in NCLEX-RN first-time test takers across the period studied suggest that bachelor's prepared candidates will slowly grow to represent an increasing proportion of test takers over time. According to the American Community Survey (ACS), approximately 44.6 percent of the nursing workforce from 2008 to 2010 held a bachelor's degree as their highest degree. In combination with the data above, this finding suggests that many nurses go on to earn additional educational degrees after beginning practice.

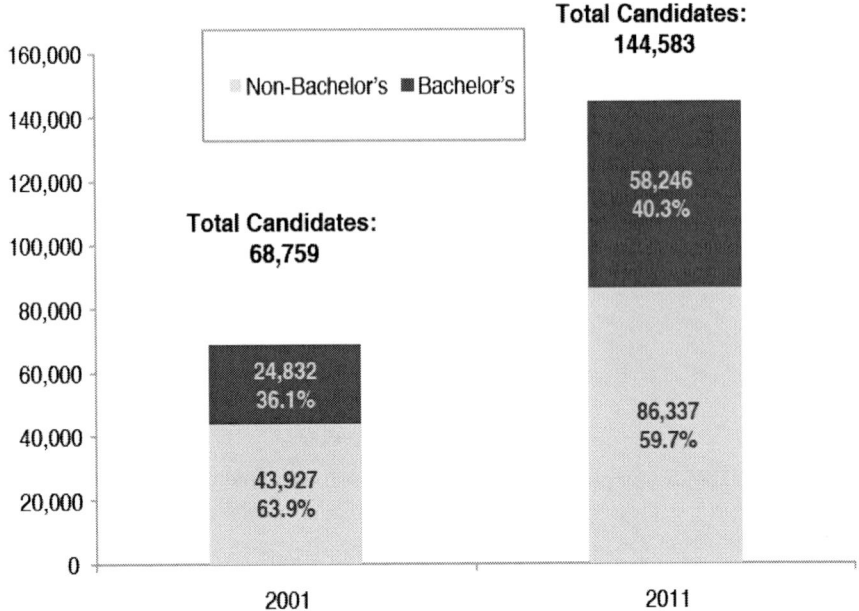

Data Source: HRSA compilation of data from the National Council of State Boards of Nursing, Nurse Licensure and NCLEX Examination Statistics Publications, 2002-2012.

Figure 20. Total Number and Percentage of NCLEX-RN First-Time Test Takers, by Bachelor's and Non-Bachelor's Degree Status, 2001 vs. 2011.

Table 9 provides first-time NCLEX candidate data, by jurisdiction of educational institution and degree attainment in 2010, the most recent year for which state-level data are available. Although candidates in a state are not necessarily converted to workers in that state, recent evidence suggests that geographic mobility among newly licensed nurses is extremely limited. [12] Therefore, it is reasonable to assume that the majority of NCLEX candidates associated with a state will in fact join that state's nursing workforce after the examination.

Table 9. NCLEX-RN First-Time Test Takers, by State and Degree Type, 2010

Jurisdiction	Diploma	Baccalaureate	Associate Degree	Total	Per Capita
Alabama	0	1,328	2,067	3,395	71.0
Alaska	0	101	88	189	26.6
Arizona	0	742	2,065	2,807	43.9
Arkansas	305	557	834	1,696	58.2
California	0	3,828	7,515	11,343	30.4
Colorado	0	984	908	1,892	37.6
Connecticut	139	655	506	1,300	36.4
Delaware	21	207	254	482	53.7
District of Columbia	0	224	83	307	51.0
Florida	0	2,211	5,350	7,561	40.2
Georgia	0	1,489	1,476	2,965	30.6
Hawaii	0	410	159	569	41.8
Idaho	0	145	481	626	39.9
Illinois	19	2,410	3,015	5,444	42.4
Indiana	44	1,709	2,328	4,081	62.9
Iowa	0	649	1,421	2,070	68.0
Kansas	0	743	1,116	1,859	65.2
Kentucky	0	853	1,879	2,732	63.0
Louisiana	37	1,317	917	2,271	50.1
Maine	0	355	308	663	49.9
Maryland	0	937	1,423	2,360	40.9
Massachusetts	66	1,779	1,486	3,331	50.9
Michigan	0	2,031	2,882	4,913	49.7
Minnesota	0	1,030	1,898	2,928	55.2
Mississippi	0	437	1,280	1,717	57.9
Missouri	63	1,831	1,517	3,411	57.0
Montana	0	215	181	396	40.0

Table 9. (Continued)

Jurisdiction	Diploma	Baccalaureate	Associate Degree	Total	Per Capita
Nebraska	0	783	387	1,170	64.1
Nevada	0	402	406	808	29.9
New Hampshire	0	211	438	649	49.3
New Jersey	701	995	1,238	2,934	33.4
New Mexico	0	275	726	1,001	48.6
New York	14	2,975	6,696	9,685	50.0
North Carolina	148	1,308	2,496	3,952	41.4
North Dakota	0	367	85	452	67.2
Ohio	319	2,868	4,719	7,906	68.5
Oklahoma	0	968	1,313	2,281	60.8
Oregon	0	686	622	1,308	34.1
Pennsylvania	1,288	2,965	2,891	7,144	56.2
Rhode Island	32	316	207	555	52.7
South Carolina	0	844	1,350	2,194	47.4
South Dakota	0	344	363	707	86.8
Tennessee	0	1,660	1,399	3,059	48.2
Texas	144	3,547	5,392	9,083	36.1
Utah	0	366	1,094	1,460	52.8
Vermont	0	102	208	310	49.5
Virginia	428	1,243	1,874	3,545	44.3
Washington	0	794	1,692	2,486	37.0
West Virginia	0	665	564	1,229	66.3
Wisconsin	0	1,455	1,679	3,134	55.1
Wyoming	0	74	279	353	62.6
Total	**3,768**	**55,390**	**81,555**	**140,713**	**45.6**

Data Source: HRSA compilation of data from the National Council of State Boards of Nursing, Nurse Licensure and NCLEX Examination Statistics Publications, 2012

Note: Total excludes NCLEX-RN candidates from the American Samoa, Guam, Northern Mariana Islands, and the Virgin Islands, which accounted for 64 first-time test takers in 2010. Total also excludes 105 Special Program Code candidates. Per capita figures for the country are based on the sum of the total graduates and the sum of the individual state populations.

Seventeen states had more bachelor's degree candidates than associate's degree candidates taking the NCLEX exam for the first time, with North Dakota leading the list with 81.2 percent BSN-educated candidates. Although the proportion of diploma-educated candidates in the national NCLEX-RN pool was small, these numbers masked a large degree of variability across the 50 U.S. states: Thirty-five states had no diploma graduate NCLEX-RN candidates, while 92 percent of the diploma graduate NCLEX-RN candidates were concentrated in eight states.

Figure 21 shows a shaded map of NCLEX-RN first-time candidates per capita. The data identify states producing more or fewer new RNs relative to their state population. Unlike the absolute pipeline figures, per capita data reveal regional variation more clearly, with all but three of the top 10 states in the Midwest region of the United States and the remainder in the South.

While per capita data suggest areas where production is higher or lower than the national average, these data do not reflect state-level differences in population characteristics, disease prevalence, or current adequacy of the nurse supply.

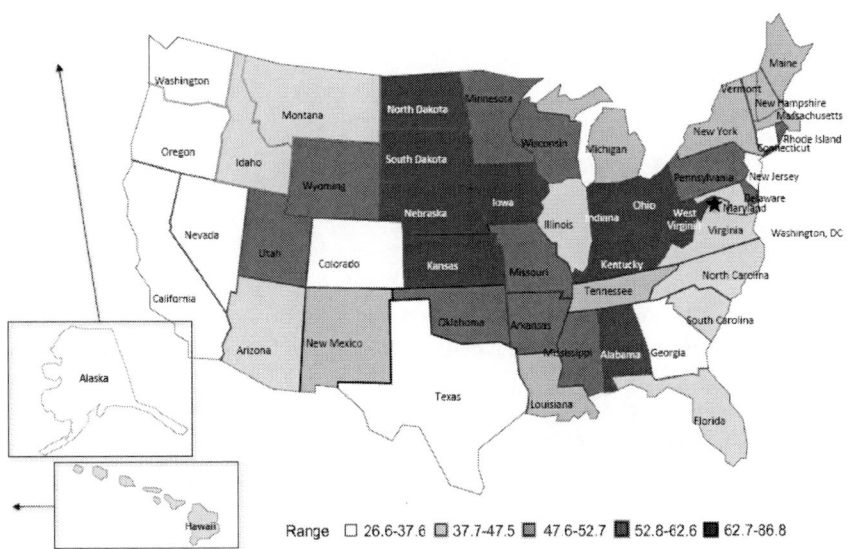

Data Source: HRSA compilation of data from the National Council of State Boards of Nursing, Nurse Licensure and NCLEX Examination Statistics Publications, 2012.

Figure 21. NCLEX-RN First-Time Test Takers per Capita, 2010.

Licensed Practical Nurses

As shown in Figure 22, the LPN pipeline, defined here as the number of individuals passing the NCLEX-PN, has grown substantially across the past decade. From 2001 to 2011, the pipeline grew from 33,448 to 60,302, an 80-percent increase. Although growth was generally consistent across the period studied, the growth rate declined slightly from 2007 to 2009. In addition, there was a surprising decrease in the number of individuals passing the NCLEX from 2010 to 2011. This finding is at least partly attributable to lower pass rates across NCLEX candidates, as well as to a decrease in the number of first-time exam takers.

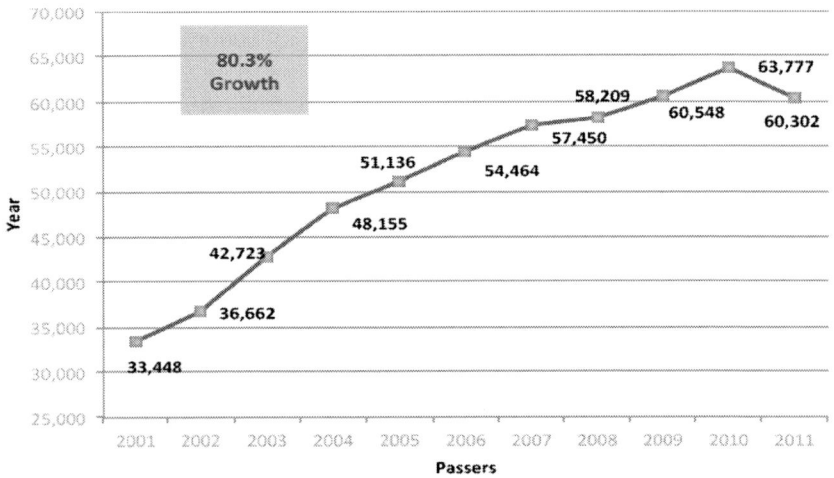

Data Source: HRSA compilation of data from the National Council of State Boards of Nursing, Nurse Licensure and NCLEX Examination Statistics Publications, 2002-2012.

Figure 22. NCLEX-PN Passers, 2001 to 2011.

Table 10 displays NCLEX-PN first-time candidates, by state, for 2010, as well as the number of candidates per capita, while Figure 23 examines the link between state population and per capita LPN candidates graphically to highlight regional trends. With the single exception of New Jersey, the top 10 states for the per capita LPN pipeline, which include Ohio, Iowa, Delaware, Arkansas, Kansas, Oklahoma, New Jersey, Minnesota, Virginia, and Louisiana, are all found in the Midwest and the South. Coastal states, including those in the Northeast and the Pacific, are generally evenly distributed across the per capita rank list.

Table 10. NCLEX-PN First-Time Test Takers, by State, 2010

State	Candidates	Candidates per Capita
Alabama	863	18.1
Alaska	19	2.7
Arizona	539	8.4
Arkansas	1,163	39.9
California	8,865	23.8
Colorado	463	9.2
Connecticut	936	26.2
Delaware	376	41.9
District of Columbia	533	88.6
Florida	4,155	22.1
Georgia	1,407	14.5
Hawaii	138	10.1
Idaho	267	17.0
Illinois	1,964	15.3
Indiana	1,453	22.4
Iowa	1,365	44.8
Kansas	990	34.7
Kentucky	1,147	26.4
Louisiana	1,354	29.9
Maine	106	8.0
Maryland	285	4.9
Massachusetts	864	13.2
Michigan	1,444	14.6
Minnesota	1,631	30.8
Mississippi	823	27.7
Missouri	1,408	23.5
Montana	131	13.2
Nebraska	472	25.8

Table 10. (Continued)

State	Candidates	Candidates per Capita
Nevada	45	1.7
New Hampshire	284	21.6
New Jersey	2,935	33.4
New Mexico	188	9.1
New York	3,586	18.5
North Carolina	1,066	11.2
North Dakota	166	24.7
Ohio	5,226	45.3
Oklahoma	1,255	33.5
Oregon	419	10.9
Pennsylvania	2,343	18.4
Rhode Island	48	4.6
South Carolina	611	13.2
South Dakota	199	24.4
Tennessee	1,706	26.9
Texas	5,629	22.4
Utah	591	21.4
Vermont	168	26.8
Virginia	2,410	30.1
Washington	1,037	15.4
West Virginia	492	26.6
Wisconsin	1,051	18.5
Wyoming	118	20.9
Total	**66,734**	**21.6**

Data Source: HRSA compilation of data from the National Council of State Boards of Nursing, Nurse Licensure and NCLEX Examination Statistics Publications, 2012
Note: Total excludes NCLEX-PN candidates from the American Samoa, Guam, Northern Mariana Islands, and the Virgin Islands, which accounted for 76 first-time test takers in 2010.

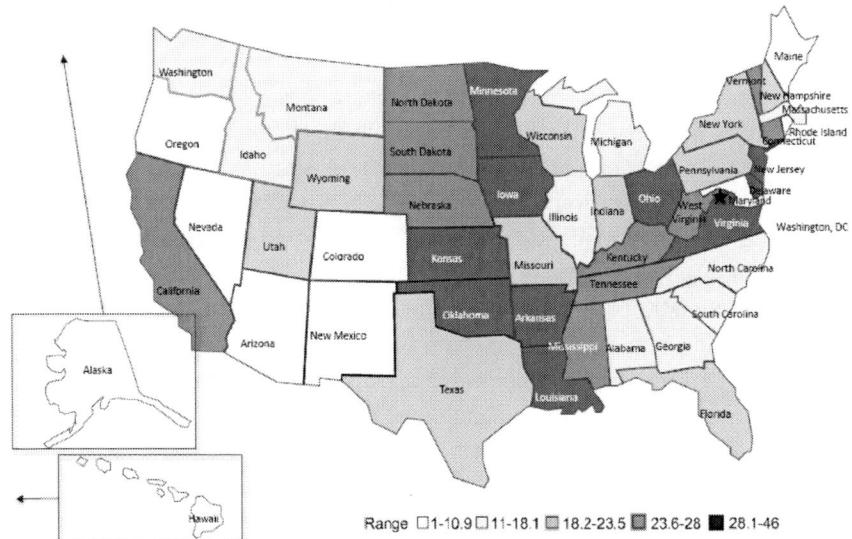

Data Source: HRSA compilation of data from the National Council of State Boards of Nursing, Nurse Licensure and NCLEX Examination Statistics Publications, 2012.

Figure 23. NCLEX-PN First-Time Test Takers per Capita, 2010.

Post-Licensure Nurse Education

While the education of a given health profession is important to the health workforce planning community, the educational progression of nurses is of particular interest given the recent recommendations for increasing the educational attainment of RNs. As noted in Section 1 of this report, the Institute of Medicine (IOM) recommended a large increase in the proportion of RNs holding a bachelor's degree. Analysis of Census Bureau data revealed that the proportion of RNs with a bachelor's or graduate degree had increased by only 5 percentage points during the 2000s, a much slower rate of growth than needed to reach the recommended 80-percent bachelor's prepared by the year 2020.

Data on NCLEX examinations showed that the proportion of candidates prepared with a BSN has increased in the past decade, but only by 3 percentage points. Increasing postlicensure RN education is another route to meeting the IOM recommendation. Although only 39 percent of pre-licensure RNs have obtained a bachelor's degree, bachelor's prepared RNs represent

44.6 percent of the RN workforce, according to the ACS data presented in Section 1.

This finding suggests that an important minority of bachelor's prepared RNs received their bachelor's degree after initial licensure. Educational data tracking the annual number of post-licensure graduates can help inform projections of the future composition of the RN workforce.

Several nursing organizations collect data on nursing program enrollments and graduations. The American Association of Colleges of Nursing (AACN) is a national association representing bachelor's and graduate nursing education at over 600 public and private universities and colleges. AACN conducts an annual survey of member and non-member universities and publishes the most current statistics available on student enrollment and graduations. Subsequent figures in this section explore data on post-licensure BSN, master's, and doctoral graduates.

About the Data

AACN annually distributes surveys requesting graduation numbers from bachelor's and higher-degree nursing education programs. This section explores results from the 2007 to 2011 surveys, which produced data for the scholastic years 2006 to 2007 through 2010 to 2011.

The 2011 to 2012 survey, which captured graduation data for the 2010 to 2011 scholastic year, was distributed to 838 institutions in September 2011 and achieved a response rate of 87.5 percent. The number of surveys distributed by AACN and the response rate achieved on these surveys vary annually.

Source: Fang, D., Li, Y., & Bednash, G. D. (2012). 2011-2012 Enrollment and Graduations in Baccalaureate and Graduate Programs in Nursing. Washington, DC: American Association of Colleges of Nursing; additional data provided upon request from AACN.

The number of RNs who graduated from post-licensure bachelor's degree programs grew from 14,946 to 27,845 from 2007 to 2011, an increase of approximately 86 percent (see Figure 24) in just four years. These "RN to BSN" graduate data indicate that RNs are increasingly advancing their education. If this growth continues, progress toward the IOM goal of increasing nurse education levels is more likely than the supply trends over the past decade (presented in Section 1) suggest is likely.

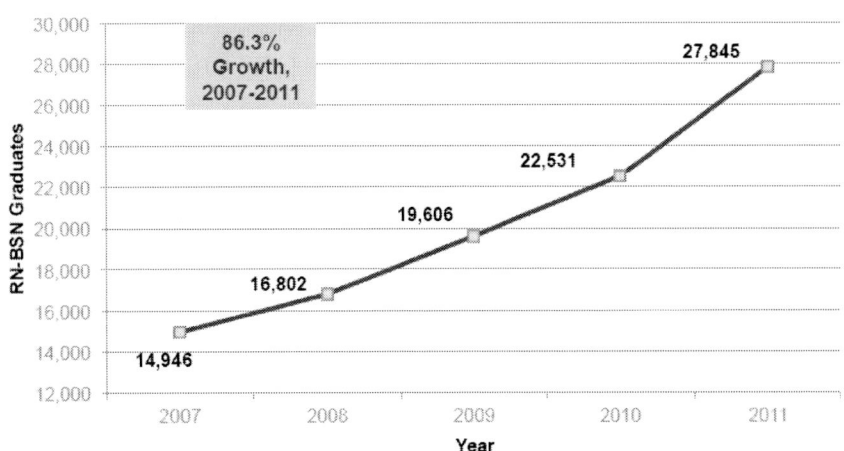

Data Source: HRSA compilation of data from the AACN Research and Data Center, 2012.

Figure 24. Licensed RNs Graduating With BSN Qualification, 2007 to 2011.

More caution is warranted when evaluating state-level post-licensure data. Many RN to BSN students are enrolled in online degree programs and therefore may live in a state other than the state where the academic program is physically located. Post-licensure graduations can be recorded by the state where the physical institution is housed, but the graduates themselves could live and work anywhere in the country. Rather than identifying states that may be underproducing, state per capita data on post-licensure graduates may more likely identify states that "export" graduates through online education. For this reason, state-level post-licensure data are not presented.

Figure 25 displays the number of master's and doctoral-prepared nurse graduates nationally from 2007 to 2011. These nurses, in addition to potentially fulfilling team leadership roles at clinical sites, serve another critical function: educating the future nursing workforce.

The annual output of master's graduates has increased by about 60 percent, while the production of doctoral graduates has more than *tripled*, over the past four years. In total, the annual number of nursing graduate degrees awarded has grown 67.4 percent.

While the growth over the course of the past four years is impressive, anecdotal and survey evidence indicates that nurse faculty shortages are a longstanding concern. In AACN's most recent survey, the national faculty vacancy rate was estimated at 7.6 percent. Therefore, almost two-thirds of the nursing schools reported faculty vacancies as a reason for not accepting all qualified applicants into the entry-level bachelor's programs.[13]

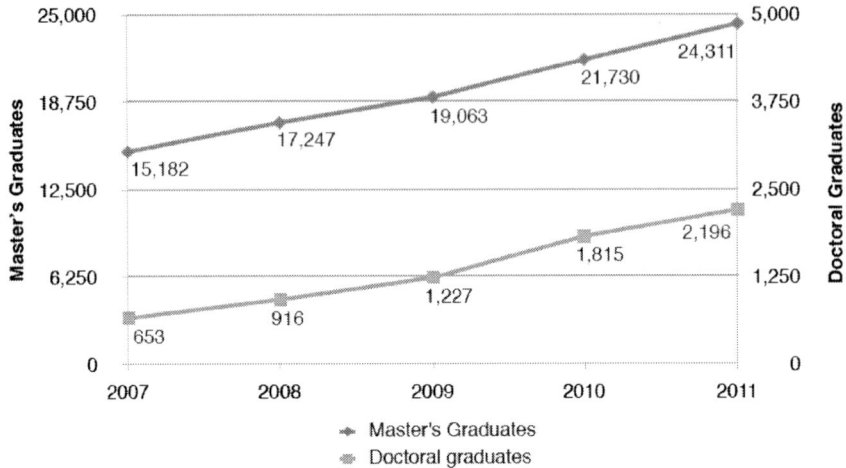

Data Source: HRSA compilation of data from the AACN Research and Data Center, 2012.

Figure 25. Master's and Doctoral Graduates, 2007 to 2011.

Advanced Clinical Roles of Special Interest

Advanced Practice Registered Nurses (APRNs), nurses who are educated at the master's or doctoral level, are of particular interest to the workforce planning community in the United States. APRNs are important providers of health care and are increasingly considered as the country faces a growing and aging population and an expansion of health insurance coverage. Both of these factors will cause increased demand for health care services, particularly primary care.

Nurse Practitioners (NPs) practice in primary care and acute care settings. NPs provide initial, ongoing, and comprehensive care for patients, including assessment, diagnosis, treatment, and management of patients with acute and chronic illnesses. While the degree of independence or supervision required by a licensed (physician) provider for the NP to practice varies with state law, NPs are widely considered a critical component of the patient care workforce.

Figure 26 shows substantial growth in the production of NPs from 2001 to 2011. In 11 years, the number of NP graduates grew from 7,261 to 12,273, a growth of approximately 69 percent.

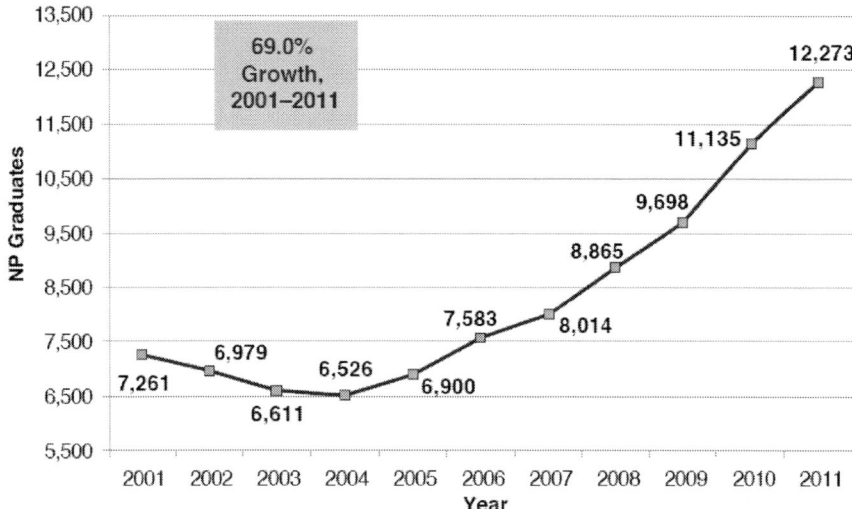

Data Source: HRSA compilation of data from the AACN Annual Survey (in collaboration with the National Organization of Nurse Practitioner Faculties for collection of nurse practitioner data) Note: Counts include master's and post-master's degree NP and NP/Clinical Nurse Specialist graduates as well as Bachelor's-to-Doctorate of Nursing Practice graduates.

Figure 26. Nurse Practitioner Graduates, 2001 to 2011.

Certified registered nurse anesthetists practice in many settings, including academic medical centers, community hospitals, outpatient surgery centers, pain clinics, or physician offices. Similar to the NP, the degree of independence or supervision needed by a licensed provider (physician, dentist, or podiatrist) for the nurse anesthetist to practice varies with state law.

Over the past 10 years, the number of nurse anesthetist graduates has increased substantially, rising from 1,159 graduates in 2001 to 2,447 graduates in 2011 (see Figure 27).

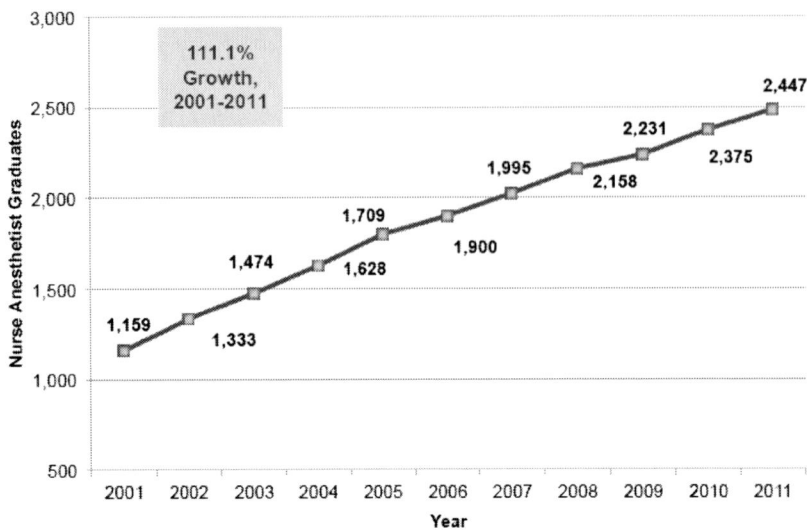

Data Source: National Board of Certification and Recertification for Nurse Anesthetists.

Figure 27. Nurse Anesthetist Graduates, 2001 to 2011.

About the Data

Data on new-entrant certified registered nurse anesthetists and certified nurse midwives were obtained from the American Association of Nurse Anesthetists (AANA) and the American Midwifery Certification Board (AMCB), respectively. Some certified registered nurse anesthetists and certified nurse midwives are educated outside of schools of nursing and are not captured in the AACN annual survey. As a result, AACN data may underestimate the total number of new-entrant certified registered nurse anesthetists and certified nurse midwives.

The AANA provided data on certified registered nurse anesthetist graduates on request. Information on the number of newly certified nurse midwives was obtained from AMCB annual reports, available at: http://www.amcbmidwife.org/c/104/about-us.

Certified nurse midwives play an important role in women's health care throughout the lifespan, providing gynecologic and perinatal care as well as other primary care services. Nurse midwives work in a variety of settings, including private offices, the offices of other health care practitioners, birth centers, hospitals, and public health.

Over the past 10 years, the number of newly certified nurse midwives has fluctuated. It declined through the early 2000s, but has rebounded in the last four years. Their number has grown from 285 newly certified nurse midwives in 2007 to nearly 400 in 2011 (see Figure 28).

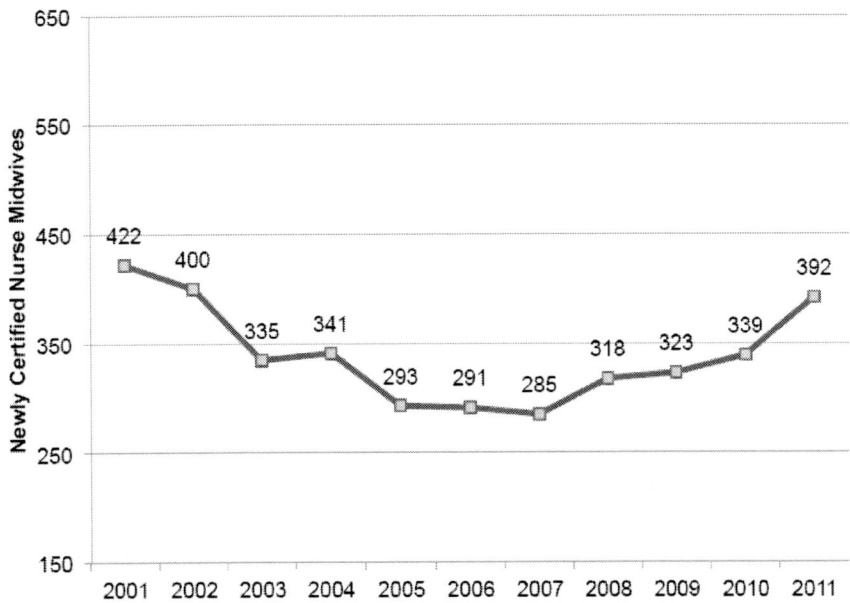

Data Source: HRSA compilation of data from the AMCB, 2010 and 2011 Annual Reports.

Figure 28. Newly Certified Nurse Midwives, 2001 to 2011.

The U.S. Nursing Pipeline and Internationally Educated Nurses

Internationally educated nurses are another source of pipeline for the U.S. nursing workforce, especially in times of shortage in domestic supply. Health workforce migration, a critical issue for many years, has received increased attention recently as a result of the 2010 World Health Organization Global Code of Practice on the International Recruitment of Health Personnel ("Global Code"). The Global Code represents an effort to promote ethical principles in the recruitment of international health personnel, with a particular focus on minimizing recruitment from countries experiencing critical shortages. Because nurse migration is a topic of interest to nursing workforce stakeholders in the United States, this section explores recent trends in internationally educated RN and LPN licensure candidates.

Identifying data sources to track the migration of internationally educated nurses into the United States is a challenge. Although some nurses may apply for visas based on their professional status as health care workers, others may enter on a spousal visa or other dependent visa, making professional visa data incomplete. Regardless of how a nurse enters the United States, however, (s)he must pass the appropriate NCLEX exam in order to be eligible for a state license (and thus, to work as a nurse). As such, the following information explores trends in internationally educated nurses who pass the appropriate NCLEX exam.

About the Data

An individual may take the NCLEX exam at a U.S. testing facility or at one of the international testing sites. International testing sites are located in Australia, Canada, England, Germany, Hong Kong, India, Japan, Mexico, the Philippines, Puerto Rico, and Taiwan. Those who seek to enter the United States on the basis of their professional status as a nurse will take the NCLEX exam prior to migrating. Others may enter the country using a different type of visa and test after their entry to the United States.

NCLEX exam data are one indicator of the overall level of interest in migrating to the United States. However, it is important to note that these data cannot differentiate those nurses who ultimately migrated from the pool of nurses who were exploring the possibility. These data therefore represent the upper limit of the number that could become licensed in the United States. They also are intended to serve only as a relative gauge for the outcome of a critical checkpoint in the process of an internationally educated nurse's journey to U.S. licensure.

The number of internationally educated NCLEX-RN passers fluctuated significantly over the past decade (see Figure 29). Steady increases in the earlier part of the decade were followed by a substantial decrease after 2007, immediately following the economic recession. U.S.educated NCLEX-RN candidates, on the other hand, experienced steady and sustained growth from 2001 to 2010, more than doubling their numbers by the end of the decade (as shown in Figure 18). These data suggest that the in-migration of internationally educated nurses may be sensitive to the effects of the macro-economic climate as well as the domestic production of nurses. There are likely to be fewer U.S. job opportunities for internationally educated nurses as a result of the doubling of domestic production over the past decade.

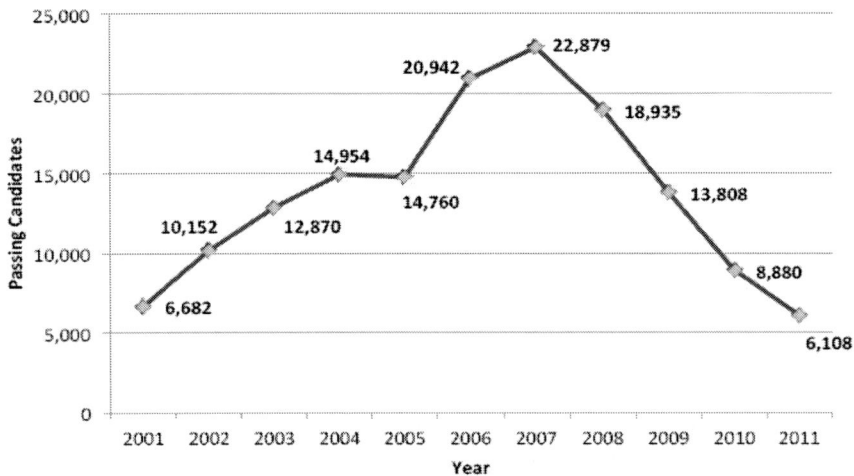

Data Source: HRSA compilation of data from the National Council of State Boards of Nursing, Nurse Licensure and NCLEX Examination Statistics Publications, 2012.

Figure 29. Internationally Educated Nurses Passing the NCLEX-RN, 2001 to 2011.

Figure 30 displays the top five countries of education for NCLEX-RN passers in 2010 and the number of individuals passing the exam from each country. With 5,188 individuals passing the NCLEX-RN, the Philippines contributed by far the highest number of individuals to the U.S. pipeline of internationally educated nurses in 2010—almost seven times that of South Korea, which ranked at number two.

In contrast to both internationally educated RNs and domestic LPNs, the international pipeline of LPNs experienced a net decline across the past decade (see Figure 31). Unlike internationally educated RNs, which showed steady growth across the early portion of the decade before declining in 2007, the internationally educated LPN pipeline experienced a second period of decline in the earlier part of the decade followed by a brief resurgence in 2006. Like internationally educated RNs, international LPN supply declined from 2007 onward. The volume of internationally educated LPNs sitting for and passing the NCLEX was, across the time period as a whole, dramatically lower than the number of RNs.

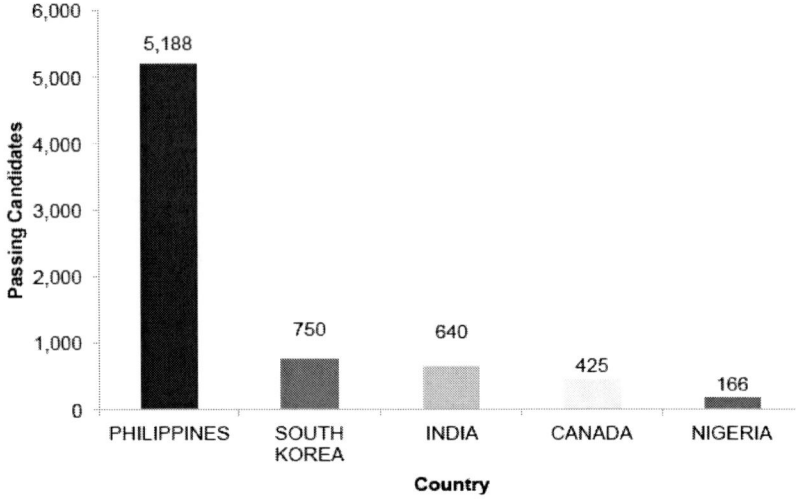

Data Source: HRSA compilation of data from the National Council of State Boards of Nursing, data provided upon request.

Figure 30. Internationally Educated Nurses Passing the NCLEX-RN, by Country, 2010.

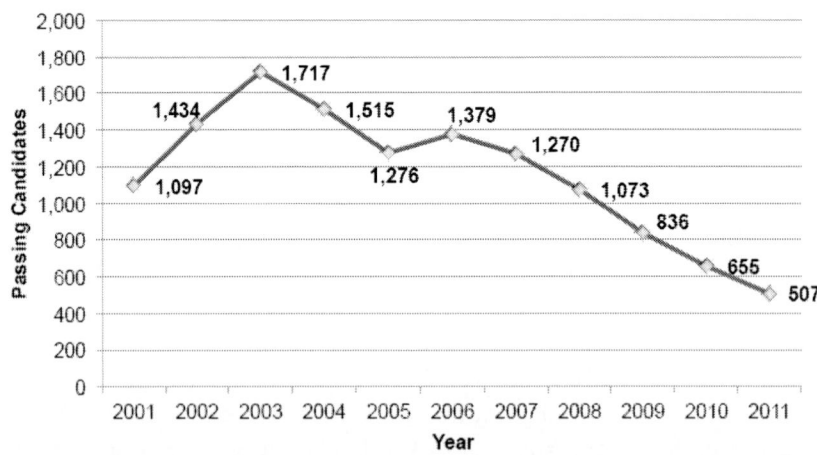

Data Source: HRSA compilation of data from the National Council of State Boards of Nursing, Nurse Licensure and NCLEX Examination Statistics Publications, 2012.

Figure 31. Internationally Educated Nurses Passing the NCLEX-PN, 2001 to 2011.

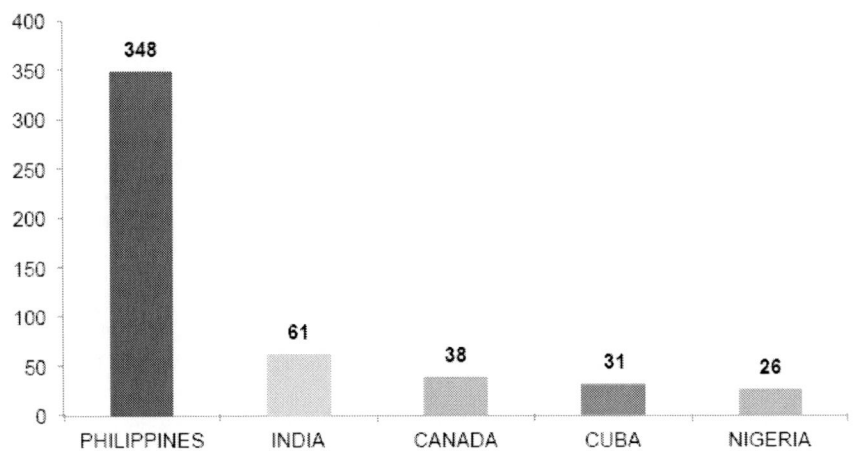

Data Source: HRSA compilation of data from the National Council of State Boards of Nursing, data provided upon request.

Figure 32. Internationally Educated Nurses Passing the NCLEX-PN, by Country, 2010.

Figure 32 displays the top five countries of education for NCLEX-PN passers in 2010 and the number of individuals passing the exam from each country. As with the NCLEX-RN, the Philippines contributed by far the highest number of individuals to the pipeline of internationally educated LPNs in 2010.

End Notes

[1] Information on the nurse supply is based on data collected by the U.S. Census Bureau: the combined American Community Survey 2008 to 2010 and the Census 2000 Long Form. The sources cover a time period of approximately one decade.

[2] Information about new entrants to the field was obtained from the National Council of State Boards of Nursing, the organization administering the RN and LPN licensure exams.

[3] Data about post-licensure education capacity was obtained from the American Association of Colleges of Nursing.

[4] The geographic unit used for this analysis is the Public Use Microdata Area (PUMA). PUMAs, the smallest geographic unit available on the ACS public use files, are areas containing 100,000 people. In this report, an "urban" PUMA is one in which a majority of residents live in metropolitan areas, as defined by the Office of Management and Budget (OMB, 2003); "rural" PUMAs are those with a majority in non-metro counties. (See http://www.whitehouse.gov/omb/bulletins_b03-04.) The classification of PUMAs as rural or urban employed a coding scheme developed by the U.S. Department of Agriculture and based on the OMB metro/non-metro classification. PUMAs represent the household

location of survey respondents. It is not possible to present a rural-urban distribution according to the work location of survey respondents.

[5] Census data report the level but not the type of degree held by individuals with less than a bachelor's degree. Therefore, RNs who reported a high school diploma or "some college, no degree" were assumed to hold an RN diploma.

[6] See http://www.iom.edu/Reports/2010/The-Future-of-Nursing-Leading-Change-Advancing-Health.aspx.

[7] See http://www.rwjf.org/content/dam/supplementary-assets

[8] See http://bhpr.hrsa.gov/healthworkforce/reports/diversityreviewevidence.pdf.

[9] The Census Bureau collects Hispanic/Latino ethnicity in a separate question from race. For this analysis, we have coded all Hispanics as "Hispanic/Latino" regardless of their selection for race.

[10] The Census Bureau uses the North American Industry Classification System (NAICS) codes for recording employment setting, and though they are limited in the level of detail available, the data sources used here offer some insights into changes in the distribution of nurses across settings.

[11] Employment distribution across settings over time was also assessed using data from the Bureau of Labor Statistics' (BLS's) Occupational Employment Statistics program. The results were generally similar, although the percentage decrease of RNs and LPNs in physicians' offices was much smaller. As a result, the BLS employment estimates do not show absolute declines in the number of RNs and LPNs in physicians' offices. The BLS data suggest that medical assistant employment growth has been rapid and that physicians' offices are becoming more heavily staffed by medical assistants.

[12] Kovner, C., Corcoran, S., & C. Brewer. (2011). "The Relative Geographic Immobility Of New Registered Nurses Calls For New Strategies To Augment That Workforce." *Health Affairs*, 30(12): 2293-2300.

[13] See http://www.aacn.nche.edu/media

In: U.S. Nursing Workforce
Editor: Marla Parris

ISBN: 978-1-63463-540-0
© 2015 Nova Science Publishers, Inc.

Chapter 2

THE U.S. NURSING WORKFORCE: TECHNICAL DOCUMENTATION[*]

National Center for Health Workforce Analysis

This technical document is a companion to the report *The U.S. Nursing Workforce: Trends in Supply and Education.*[1] It provides additional information on data and methodology for analysis of the nurse supply, including information on the calculation of standard errors, tests of significance for change over time, and use of the data for rural-urban analysis.

DATA SOURCES FOR ANALYSIS OF THE NURSE SUPPLY

Data from Census 2000 and the American Community Survey were used to analyze the nurse supply over a period of approximately one decade. The 2000 Census data file was obtained from the Integrated Public Use Microdata Series (IPUMS)-USA maintained at the Minnesota Population Center at the University of Minnesota.[2] The 2000 Census data are a 5 percent national random sample of the population that completed the Census long form.[3] The 2000 Census sample file has 14,081,466 records.

---

[*] This is an edited, reformatted and augmented version of a report issued by the Health Resources and Services Administration, U.S. Department of Health and Human Services, October 2013.

The American Community Survey (ACS) Public Use Microdata Sample (PUMS) data were downloaded from the U.S. Census Bureau.[4] The 2008-2010 ACS data file is an approximately 3 percent sample of the U.S. population constructed by combining the 1 percent samples in the 2008, 2009, and 2010 ACS. There are 9,093,077 records in the 3-year 2008-2010 ACS data file. The 3-year ACS file was used, rather than the most recent single-year ACS file, in order to have sufficient sample sizes for state-level analysis and multi-variable cross tabulations.

The 2000 Census represents a single year in which data were collected between about March and July of 2000. The ACS data are collected throughout each calendar year and represent the aggregate characteristics over a 3-year period.

STANDARD ERROR CALCULATION FOR CENSUS 2000 SAMPLE DATA

The standard errors of 2000 estimates were calculated using the design factor method outlined in documentation from the U.S. Census Bureau.[5] The design factor represents the effects of the sample design and estimation procedure used for the Census 2000 sample data. The Census long form public use data file does not contain variables for the parameters of the complex sample design or replicate weights for direct estimation of standard errors. In general, the design factor method provides a conservative estimate of standard errors.

In the calculation of a standard error in the Census 2000 sample, first the unadjusted standard error is calculated. Then the unadjusted standard error is multiplied by the design factor for the characteristic. For example, the design factor for race is 2.2, and that for sex is 1.2.[4]

The formula for calculating the unadjusted standard error (SE) of a percent in the Census 2000 sample is:

$$SE(p) = \sqrt{\left[\frac{19}{B}\right] p(100-p)}$$

where p = the percent and B = the estimated (weighted) base or denominator used in calculating the percent.[4] The result from this formula is multiplied by the design factor to derive the approximate adjusted standard error.

STANDARD ERROR CALCULATION FOR 2008-2010 AMERICAN COMMUNITY SURVEY PUMS DATA

The 2008-2010 3-year ACS PUMS file contains 80 replicate weights for direct calculation of standard errors. As stated in documentation for 2008-2010 3-year ACS:[6]

> The standard error of X can be computed after the replicate estimates X1 through X80 are computed [using each replicate weight]. The standard error is estimated using the sum of squared differences between each replicate estimate Xr and the full sample estimate X.

The standard error (SE) formula using replicate weights is:

$$SE(X) = \sqrt{\left(\frac{4}{80}\right) \sum_{r=1}^{80} (X_r - X)^2}$$

In the SUDAAN statistical software package, there are two methods of calculating standard errors using replicate weights: (1) the jackknife method and (2) balance repeated replication (BRR). Using BRR for the formula above, the code for a crosstab procedure is:[7]

proc crosstab data=[name] design = BRR;
weight pwgtp;
repwgt pwgtp1-pwgtp80 / adjfay = 4;

where pwgtp is the name of the person weight variable in the ACS data file and pwgtp1-pwtp80 are the names of the respective replicate weight variables. The statement "adjfay=4" adjusts for the "4/80" in the formula. Either the jackknife or BRR method can be used, with the relevant specified adjustment, as each produced the same standared errors.[8] The replicate weights in the ACS can have a negative value. SUDAAN treats negative replicate weights as zero.

The significance of the differences between 2000 and 2008-2010 were based upon the Z value calculated from the following formula:[9]

$$Z = \frac{A - B}{\sqrt{[SE(A)]^2 + [SE(B)]^2}}$$

A is the percent in 2008-2010 and B is the percent in 2000. Differences are reported as statistically significant if $p < .05$, i.e., $Z<-1.96$ or $Z>1.96$.

USE OF THE ACS PUMS DATA FOR RURAL-URBAN ANALYSES

The American Community Survey (ACS) public-use data files do not contain a variable to indicate the metropolitan status (e.g., rural or urban) of the household location of an individual. The PUMS files do contain a geographical variable to indicate the Public Use Microdata Area (PUMA) in which a household is located. A PUMA is an area with a minimum population of 100,000. Smaller geographical units are not provided in ACS PUMS files in order to protect the confidentiality of respondents in the survey. PUMAs are defined every ten years in conjunction with the decennial census survey.[10]

The Economic Research Service at the U.S. Department of Agriculture (USDA) has constructed a classification of PUMAs as metropolitan or nonmetropolitan. This classification was applied in the analysis presented in this report.[11] The term "urban" is used for the PUMAs classified as metropolitan and the term "rural" is used for the PUMAs the USDA scheme labels as nonmetropolitan.

PUMAs can be comprised of multiple counties or subparts of a county. The USDA classified each county or county subpart in a PUMA as either metropolitan or nonmetropolitan using the USDA 2003 Rural Urban Continuum Codes (RUCC).[12] The values of the RUCC are 1 through 9 in which metropolitan counties were defined as those with RUCC values of 1, 2, or 3. All other counties were defined as nonmetropolitan.

For each county or subpart county in a PUMA, the population (in 2000) was obtained by USDA from state-level data files from the Census Bureau. The total population in a PUMA was thus divided into the number in metropolitan counties (based upon the RUCC scheme) and the number in nonmetropolitan counties. There were 1596 PUMAs (77%) where all of the population lived in metropolitan counties. In 225 PUMAs (11%), the population all lived in a nonmetropolitan county. The remaining 250 PUMAs

(12%) contained both metropolitan and nonmetropolitan counties. If over 50 percent of the total population in a PUMA was attributed to metropolitan counties making up the PUMA, then the PUMA was classified as a metropolitan area. If half or less of the PUMA population was in metropolitan counties, then the PUMA was classified as nonmetropolitan.

End Notes

[1] Available on the web at: http://bhpr.hrsa.gov/healthworkforce/index.html

[2] Steven Ruggles, J. Trent Alexander, Katie Genadek, Ronald Goeken, Matthew B. Schroeder, and Matthew Sobek. Integrated Public Use Microdata Series (IPUM): Version 5.0 [Machine-readable database]. Minneapolis: University of Minnesota, 2010. The data file from IPUM is a national data file that combines the individual state data files available from the U.S. Census Bureau (http://www2.census.gov/census_2000/datasets/PUMS/).

[3] U.S. Census Bureau. Technical Documentation: Public Use Microdata Sample, 2000 Census of Population and Housing. Washington, DC: U.S Government Printing Office; October 2008 (http://www.census.gov/prod/cen2000/doc/pums.pdf).

[4] U.S. Census Bureau at http://www2.census.gov/acs2010_3yr/pums/. See U.S. Census Bureau. A Compass for Understanding and Using American Community Survey Data: What PUMS Data Users Need to Know. Washington, DC: U.S. Government Printing Office; February 2009 (http://www.census.gov/acs/www/guidance_for_data_users/handbooks/).

[5] U.S. Census Bureau. Chapter 4: Accuracy of the Microdata Sample Estimates and Table E: Census 2000 PUMS Standard Error Design Factors—United States in Technical Documentation: Public Use Microdata Sample, 2000 Census of Population and Housing. Washington, DC: U.S Government Printing Office; October 2008 (http://www.census.gov/prod/cen2000/doc/pums.pdf).

[6] U.S. Census Bureau. 2008-2010 PUMS Accuracy of the Data. http://www.census.gov/acs/www/Downloads/data_documentation/pums/Accuracy/2008_2010AccuracyPUMS.pdf

[7] See U.S. Census Bureau. Estimating ASEC Variances with Replicate Weights. Available at the link "Estimating ASEC Variances with Replicate Weights" on the web page at http://usa.ipums.org/usa/repwt.shtml.

[8] The SUDAAN setup for the jackknife method is: "proc crosstab data=[name] design = jackknife; weight pwgtp; jackwgts pwgtp1-pwgtp80 / adjjack = .05;". The "adjjack = .05" is the adjustment for the "4/80" in the standard error formula for the ACS using replicate weights [4/80 = .05]. (See jackknife example at http://usa.ipums.org/usa/repwt.shtml.) The differences in the adjustments used for jackknife and BRR relates to the different formulas used in jackknife and BRR for calculating standard errors (see Research Triangle Institute. SUDAAN Language Manual, Release 9.0, 2004, pp. 59-62). We calculated standard errors using BRR and jackknife in SUDAAN to compare resulting standard errors. BRR (using adjfay=4) and jackknife (using adjjack = .05) produced identical standard errors in the analysis using the 2008-2010 ACS presented in this report.

[9] U.S. Census Bureau. Instructions for Applying Statistical Testing for the 2008-2010 3-Year Data and the 2006- 2010 ACS 5-Year Data. http://www.census.gov/acs/www/Downloads/data_documentation/Statistical_Testing/2010StatisticalTesting3and5year.pdf

[10] See A Compass for Understanding and Using ACS Data: What PUMS Data Users Need to Know, U.S. Census Bureau, February 2009, http://www.census.gov/acs/www/Downloads/handbooks/ACSPUMS.pdf

[11] The data file containing the USDA classification of PUMAs as metropolitan or nonmetropolitan was obtained by the Health Resources and Services Administration from USDA in September 2012 along with the paper describing the USDA method authored by Tom Hertz at USDA entitled, "Mapping County Typology Codes and Metro Status onto the Census Public Use Microdata Areas (PUMAs)."

[12] For information on the RUCC scheme see http://www.ers.usda.gov/data-products/rural-urban-continuumcodes.aspx

INDEX

A

access, vii, 1, 25
adjustment, 61, 63
advanced practice RNs, 1
African Americans, 25, 26, 27
age, 2, 4, 6, 22, 24, 26, 27, 31, 35
aging population, 22, 50
American Samoa, 42, 46
assessment, 50
assets, 58

B

base, 60
birth center, 53
Bureau of Labor Statistics, 58

C

candidates, 3, 36, 37, 38, 39, 40, 42, 43, 44, 46, 47, 54
category a, 17, 20
Census, 4, 5, 6, 20, 21, 22, 23, 24, 25, 26, 27, 28, 29, 30, 31, 32, 33, 34, 35, 47, 57, 58, 59, 60, 62, 63, 64
chronic illness, 50
cities, 9
classification, 57, 62, 64
climate, 55
coding, 57
collaboration, 51
colleges, 20, 48
community, 4, 47, 50, 51
compilation, 38, 39, 40, 42, 43, 44, 46, 47, 49, 50, 51, 53, 55, 56, 57
composition, 4, 5, 48
confidentiality, 62
covering, 4

D

database, 63
dentist, 51
Department of Agriculture, 62
Department of Health and Human Services, 1, 59
distribution, vii, 1, 2, 5, 13, 22, 24, 26, 39, 58
District of Columbia, 9

E

economic downturn, 37
Economic Research Service, 62
education, 1, 4, 22, 36, 37, 47, 48, 49, 55, 57
educational attainment, 4, 5, 37, 38, 47
educators, 1, 4

employees, 31
employers, 25
employment, 1, 4, 16, 35, 58
employment growth, 58
England, 54
enrollment, 37
ethnic groups, 27
ethnicity, 4, 25, 26, 58
evidence, 40, 49
examinations, 47

F

formula, 60, 61, 63

G

Germany, 54
growth, 2, 3, 4, 5, 20, 21, 24, 27, 31, 37, 38, 39, 44, 47, 48, 49, 51, 54, 55
growth rate, 21, 44
guidance, 63

H

health, vii, 1, 3, 4, 9, 20, 25, 28, 29, 31, 47, 50, 52, 53, 54
health care, vii, 1, 3, 20, 25, 28, 29, 31, 50, 52, 54
health care system, vii, 1, 3
health insurance, 50
health practitioners, 31
health services, 9
high school, 58
high school diploma, 58
hiring, 22
Hispanics, 25, 26, 27, 58
Hong Kong, 54

I

independence, 50, 51
India, 54

individuals, 2, 3, 5, 37, 38, 39, 44, 55, 57, 58
inflation, 35
institutions, 48
Iowa, 44
issues, 38

J

Japan, 54
jurisdiction, 37, 40

L

Latinos, 26, 27
leadership, 24, 49
level of education, 3
licensed practical nurse, vii, 5
light, 38
Louisiana, 44
LPN, vii, 1, 2, 3, 4, 6, 9, 11, 13, 14, 18, 20, 26, 27, 29, 31, 33, 44, 54, 55, 57
LPN workforce, 2, 6, 20, 27, 31

M

majority, 2, 3, 13, 17, 20, 28, 30, 32, 33, 36, 39, 40, 57
management, 50
media, 58
medical, 9, 51, 58
methodology, vii, 59
metropolitan areas, 57
Mexico, 54
migration, 53, 54, 55
Minneapolis, 63
minorities, 25, 27

N

North America, 58
nurse licensing exams, 2
nurse supply, vii, 4, 5, 22, 36, 43, 57, 59

Index

nurses, vii, 1, 2, 4, 5, 9, 13, 17, 20, 22, 24, 25, 27, 28, 30, 31, 32, 33, 36, 37, 38, 39, 40, 47, 49, 50, 53, 54, 55, 58
nursing, 1, 2, 3, 4, 5, 6, 9, 16, 21, 22, 24, 25, 28, 29, 30, 31, 35, 36, 37, 38, 39, 40, 48, 49, 50, 52, 53
nursing care, 16, 28, 29, 31
nursing home, 30
nursing workforce, 1, 2, 4, 5, 6, 9, 21, 24, 25, 36, 39, 40, 49, 53

O

Office of Management and Budget (OMB), 57
officials, 4
Oklahoma, 44
opportunities, 55
outpatient, 2, 28, 29, 31, 51

P

Pacific, 45
pain, 51
patient care, 50
perinatal, 52
Philippines, 54, 55, 57
physicians, 31, 58
pipeline, vii, 1, 2, 3, 4, 36, 38, 39, 43, 44, 53, 55, 57
policy, 1, 4
policy makers, 1, 4
population, 2, 5, 6, 11, 13, 17, 20, 21, 25, 26, 27, 30, 32, 33, 43, 44, 59, 60, 62
principles, 53
public health, 17, 20, 30, 32, 33, 53
Puerto Rico, 54
PUMA, 57, 62

R

race, 4, 25, 26, 27, 58, 60
rate of change, 22
recession, 3, 31, 54

recommendations, 47
recovery, 4, 24
reform, 4
registered nurse, vii, 1, 4, 5, 51, 52
replication, 61
researchers, 1, 4
Residential, 16, 18
response, 48
retirement, 24, 31
retirement age, 24
RN, vii, 1, 2, 3, 4, 6, 7, 9, 12, 16, 17, 20, 21, 22, 24, 25, 26, 30, 31, 32, 36, 37, 38, 39, 40, 41, 42, 43, 47, 48, 49, 54, 55, 56, 57, 58
RN workforce, 2, 9, 20, 22, 26, 31, 48
rural areas, 2, 13, 16, 22

S

sample design, 60
savings, 31
school, 36, 50, 52
services, 28, 29, 31, 50, 52
sex, 25, 60
shape, 4
shortage, 35, 53
showing, 6
software, 61
South Dakota, 6
South Korea, 55
stability, 24
staffing, 22
stakeholders, 54
standard error, vii, 5, 9, 59, 60, 61, 63
state(s), 1, 4, 5, 6, 9, 11, 40, 42, 43, 44, 49, 50, 51, 54, 60, 62, 63
statistics, 48
structure, 22, 24
student enrollment, 48
supervision, 50, 51

T

Taiwan, 54

techniques, 5
technologies, 22
testing, 5, 54
time periods, 23
treatment, 50

U

U.S. Department of Agriculture (USDA), 57, 62
United, 3, 4, 36, 38, 43, 50, 54, 63
United States, 3, 4, 36, 38, 43, 50, 54, 63
universities, 20, 48
urban, vii, 4, 5, 13, 16, 17, 20, 57, 59, 62, 64
urban areas, 5, 13, 16
USA, 59
USDA, 62, 64

V

vacancies, 50
variables, 60, 61

W

Washington, 48, 63
web, 63
workers, 31, 40, 54
workforce, 1, 2, 4, 5, 6, 9, 20, 21, 22, 24, 25, 26, 27, 29, 31, 35, 36, 38, 39, 40, 47, 48, 49, 50, 53
World Health Organization, 53

Y

young people, 24